Mental Health
Nursing
at a Glance

This title is also available as an e-book.
For more details, please see
www.wiley.com/buy/9781118465288
or scan this QR code:

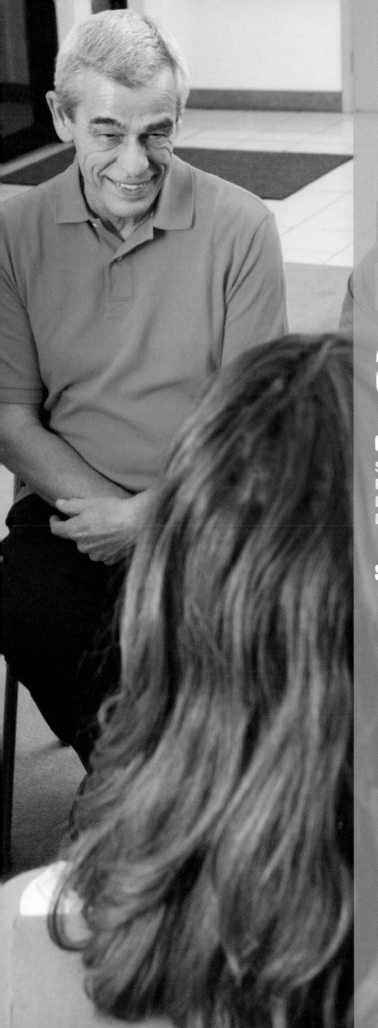

Mental Health Nursing

at a Glance

Grahame Smith

Subject Head – Allied Health
Faculty of Education, Health and Community
Liverpool John Moores University
Liverpool

Series Editor: Ian Peate

WILEY Blackwell

This edition first published 2015 © 2015 by John Wiley & Sons, Ltd.

Registered Office
John Wiley & Sons, Ltd, The Atrium, Southern Gate, Chichester, West Sussex, PO19 8SQ, UK

Editorial Offices
9600 Garsington Road, Oxford, OX4 2DQ, UK
The Atrium, Southern Gate, Chichester, West Sussex, PO19 8SQ, UK
350 Main Street, Malden, MA 02148-5020, USA

For details of our global editorial offices, for customer services and for information about how to apply for permission to reuse the copyright material in this book please see our website at www.wiley.com/wiley-blackwell

Library of Congress Cataloging-in-Publication Data

Smith, Grahame, author.
  Mental health nursing at a glance / Grahame Smith.
     p. ; cm. – (At a glance series)
  Includes bibliographical references and index.
  ISBN 978-1-118-46528-8 (pbk.)
  I. Title.   II. Series: At a glance series (Oxford, England)
  [DNLM: 1. Mental Disorders–nursing.   2. Mental Disorders–psychology.
3. Psychiatric Nursing–methods.   WY 160]
  RC440
  616.89′0231–dc23

2014005237

A catalogue record for this book is available from the British Library.

Wiley also publishes its books in a variety of electronic formats. Some content that appears in print may not be available in electronic books.

Cover image: iStock: © asiseeit
Cover design by Meaden Creative

Set in 9.5/11.5pt Minion by SPi Publisher Services, Pondicherry, India
Printed and bound in Malaysia by Vivar Printing Sdn Bhd

1   2015

Contents

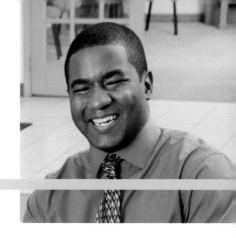

How to use your revision guide vii
About the companion website x
Introduction xii
Practice tree example xiv

Part 1 | **Essential skills 1**

1 Care, compassion and communication 2
2 Building therapeutic relationships 4
3 Values-based practice 6
4 Managing clinical risk 8
5 Infection prevention and control 10
6 Nutrition and fluid management 12
7 Elimination 14
8 Clinical observations 16
9 Documentation 18
10 Medicines management 20

Part 2 | **Nursing individuals with mental health needs 23**

11 Assessment 24
12 Risk 26
13 Classification 28
14 Psychological interventions 31
15 Schizophrenia 34
16 Depression 36
17 Bipolar affective disorder 38
18 Anxiety 40
19 Eating disorders 42
20 Personality disorders 44
21 Learning disabilities and mental health 46
22 Functional disorders in older adults 48
23 Dementia 50
24 Acute confusional states 52
25 Drug and alcohol misuse 54
26 Children and adolescent mental health 56
27 Recovery 58
28 Physical wellbeing 60
29 Mental health law 62
30 Medication and ECT 66

Part 3 **Leadership skills** **71**

31 Organising care 72
32 Leadership 74
33 Managing people 76
34 Time management 78
35 Decision-making 80
36 Utilising research 82
37 Reflection 84
38 Lifelong learning 86

Appendix: Clinical procedures 88
References and bibliography 92
Glossary 93
Index 95

How to use your revision guide

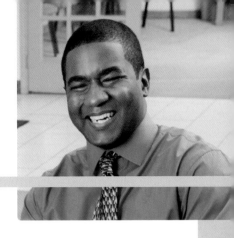

Features contained within your revision guide

Each topic is presented in a double-page spread with clear, easy-to-follow diagrams supported by succinct explanatory text.

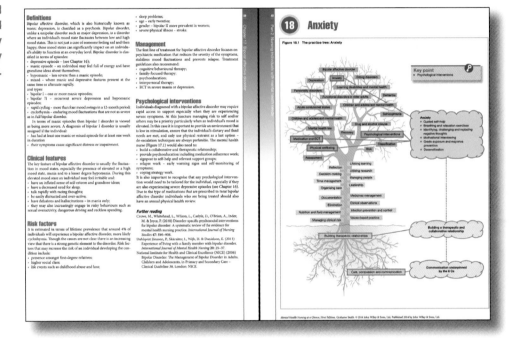

Key learning points highlight important things to remember.

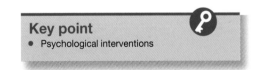

The website icon indicates that you can find accompanying resources on the book's companion website.

The anytime, anywhere textbook

Wiley E-Text

Your book is also available to purchase as a **Wiley E-Text: Powered by VitalSource** version – a digital, interactive version of this book which you own as soon as you download it.

Your **Wiley E-Text** allows you to:

Search: Save time by finding terms and topics instantly in your book, your notes, even your whole library (once you've downloaded more textbooks)

Note and Highlight: Colour code, highlight and make digital notes right in the text so you can find them quickly and easily

Organize: Keep books, notes and class materials organized in folders inside the application

Share: Exchange notes and highlights with friends, classmates and study groups

Upgrade: Your textbook can be transferred when you need to change or upgrade computers

Link: Link directly from the page of your interactive textbook to all of the material contained on the companion website

The **Wiley E-Text** version will also allow you to copy and paste any photograph or illustration into assignments, presentations and your own notes.

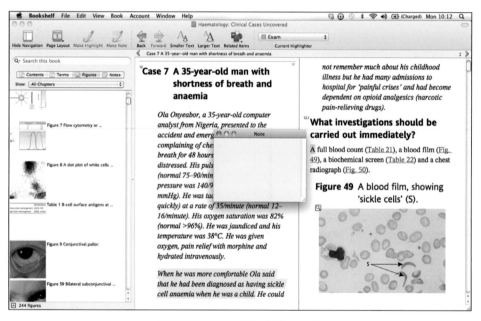

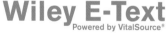
Powered by VitalSource®

To access your Wiley E-Text:

- Visit **www.vitalsource.com/software/bookshelf/downloads** to download the Bookshelf application to your computer, laptop, tablet or mobile device.

- Open the Bookshelf application on your computer and register for an account.

- Follow the registration process.

CourseSmart

CourseSmart gives you instant access (via computer or mobile device) to this Wiley-Blackwell e-book and its extra electronic functionality, at 40% off the recommended retail print price. See all the benefits at: **www.coursesmart.com/students**

Instructors … receive your own digital desk copies!
CourseSmart also offers instructors an immediate, efficient, and environmentally-friendly way to review this book for your course.

For more information visit **www.coursesmart.com/instructors**.

With CourseSmart, you can create lecture notes quickly with copy and paste, and share pages and notes with your students. Access your **Course Smart** digital book from your computer or mobile device instantly for evaluation, class preparation, and as a teaching tool in the classroom.

Simply sign in at **http://instructors.coursesmart.com/bookshelf** to download your Bookshelf and get started. To request your desk copy, hit 'Request Online Copy' on your search results or book product page.

We hope you enjoy using your new book. Good luck with your studies!

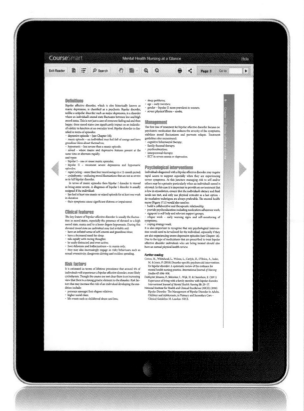

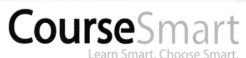

About the companion website

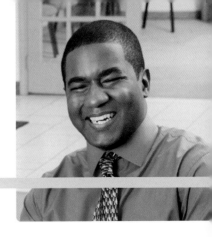

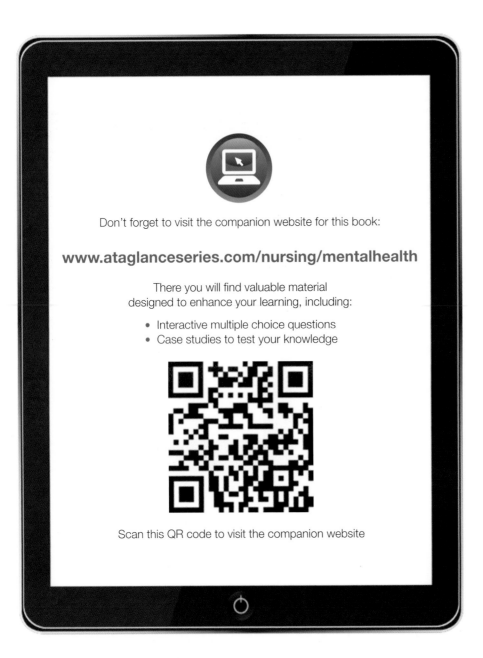

Don't forget to visit the companion website for this book:

www.ataglanceseries.com/nursing/mentalhealth

There you will find valuable material
designed to enhance your learning, including:

- Interactive multiple choice questions
- Case studies to test your knowledge

Scan this QR code to visit the companion website

Introduction

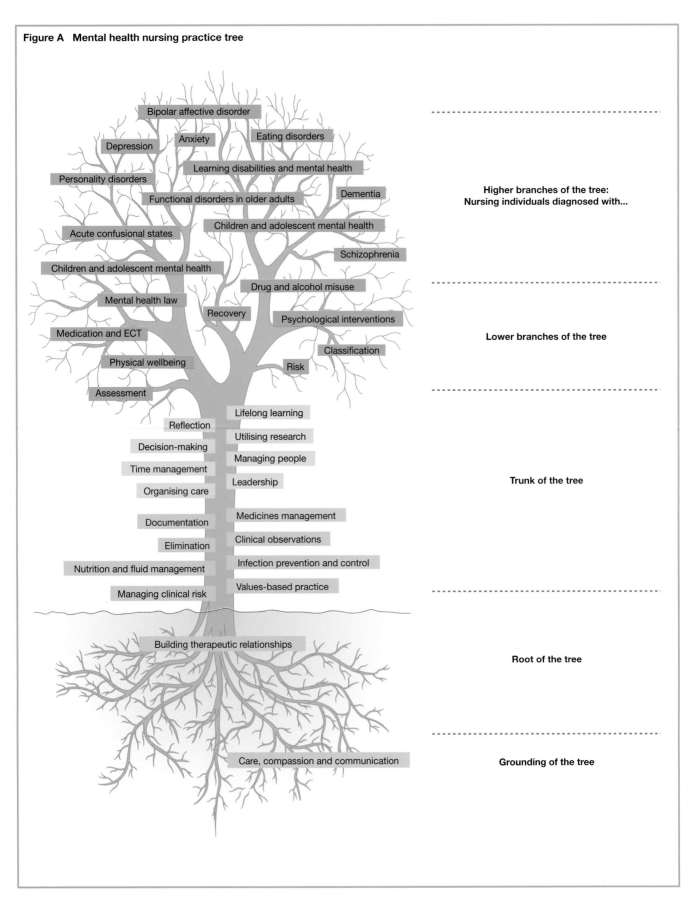

Figure A   Mental health nursing practice tree

Bipolar affective disorder

Depression

Anxiety

Eating disorders

Learning disabilities and mental health

Personality disorders

Functional disorders in older adults

Dementia

Acute confusional states

Children and adolescent mental health

Schizophrenia

Children and adolescent mental health

Drug and alcohol misuse

Mental health law

Recovery

Medication and ECT

Psychological interventions

Physical wellbeing

Classification

Risk

Assessment

Lifelong learning

Reflection

Utilising research

Decision-making

Managing people

Time management

Leadership

Organising care

Documentation

Medicines management

Elimination

Clinical observations

Nutrition and fluid management

Infection prevention and control

Managing clinical risk

Values-based practice

Building therapeutic relationships

Care, compassion and communication

Higher branches of the tree:
Nursing individuals diagnosed with...

Lower branches of the tree

Trunk of the tree

Root of the tree

Grounding of the tree

Aim

This book is written with pre-registration mental health nursing students in mind, as a "revision or notes" text. It is also designed to be a "refresher" text for registered mental health nurses. The structure of each chapter is intended to support the student's learning journey; the chapters are also explicitly underpinned by the Nursing and Midwifery Council's (NMC's) (2010) Standards for Pre-registration Nursing Education. As befits an *at a Glance* publication each chapter is a concise summary of the subject being explored, which then links to an illustrative example or "key learning point" (highlighted by a key symbol). By presenting both textual and visual information this supports different types of learners. The "Further reading" section in each chapter and the Reference list at the end of the book signpost the reader to more comprehensive information.

Professional context

The NMC's (2010) Standards for Pre-registration Nursing Education aim to:

.... enable nurses to give and support high quality care in rapidly changing environments. They reflect how future services are likely to be delivered, acknowledge future public health priorities and address the challenges of long-term conditions, an ageing population, and providing more care outside hospitals. Nurses must be equipped to lead, delegate, supervise and challenge other nurses and healthcare professionals. They must be able to develop practice, and promote and sustain change. As graduates they must be able to think analytically, use problem-solving approaches and evidence in decision-making, keep up with technical advances and meet future expectations.

(*Nursing and Midwifery Council, 2010: pp. 4–5*)

Further to this aim the NMC (2010) expect that a pre-registration nursing student by the end of their training will be competent and possess the required knowledge, skills and attitudes. These requirements are set out in a competency framework for each field of nursing, which is organised into four domains:

- professional values;
- communication and interpersonal skills;
- nursing practice and decision-making;
- leadership, management and team working.

Each domain highlights the competencies the student is expected to achieve by end of their training; each chapter will provide a summary of these domain competencies.

Structure

The book is divided into three parts with 38 corresponding chapters that link into a "practice tree" approach:

- Part 1 – Essential skills
- Part 2 – Nursing individuals with mental health needs
- Part 3 – Leadership skills

The practice tree

Mental health nurses on a day-to-day basis have to ensure that the practice decisions they make lead to positive care outcomes. This process has to be reasoned, it also has to be in partnership with service users, carers and other professionals. Having the skills to work in this way does not happen overnight; it is a process that is engendered throughout a student's pre-registration nurse training and continues throughout the registered nurse's lifelong learning journey. The focus of this book is to assist this process by using a consistent theme – **the mental health nursing practice tree**; this approach provides an illustrative guide of the reasoned decision-making process.

Pre-registration nurse training according to the NMC's (2010) standards describes skills, knowledge and attitudes as being either generic or field specific:

Generic competency relates to the knowledge, skills and attitudes and technical abilities required of all nurses by the end of a pre-registration nursing programme.

Field competency encompasses the knowledge, skills and attitudes that nurses must acquire which together with the generic competencies must have been demonstrated in order to practise in a specific field of nursing. Learning outcomes for each field are derived from both generic and field-specific competencies.

(*Nursing and Midwifery Council, 2010: p. 147*)

These different types of competencies complement each other and ensure that at the point of registration a nurse has a holistic set of competencies that they can apply in many different contexts. On this basis the practice tree (see Figure A) as an illustrative tool provides the student with a series of opportunities to explore how their requisite skills, knowledge and attitudes should be holistically developed.

The practice tree has to grow on firm ground. This relates to the use of effective communications skills underpinned by the "6 Cs". The roots of the tree and the root of effective mental health nursing practice correspond to the building of a strong therapeutic relationship that is partnership focused. Both the grounding and the roots of the practice tree are generic skills. The trunk of the tree encapsulates the further development of these generic skills and corresponds to parts 1 and 3. Field-specific skills are articulated throughout the branches of the tree and correspond to part 2. Each chapter then provides an illustrative "key learning point" or "chapter cloud", which demonstrates how these specific skills link to the practice tree.

It is important to recognise that the practice tree is an illustrative example and that the student nurse should apply both generic and field competencies in an integrated and fluid way, and under the supervision of their mentor.

Practice tree example

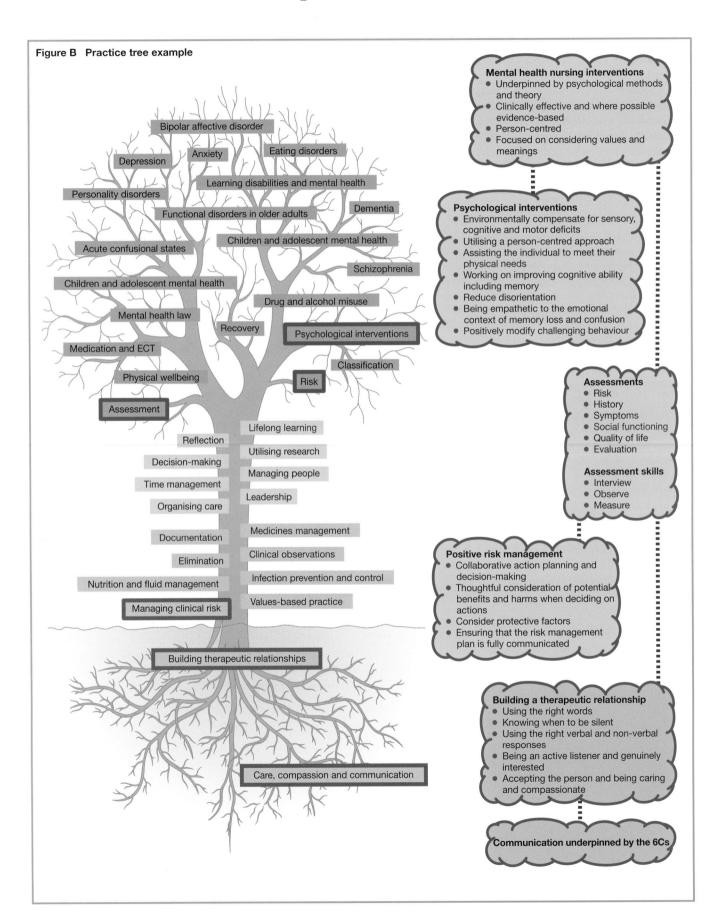

Figure B   Practice tree example

Mental health nursing interventions
- Underpinned by psychological methods and theory
- Clinically effective and where possible evidence-based
- Person-centred
- Focused on considering values and meanings

Psychological interventions
- Environmentally compensate for sensory, cognitive and motor deficits
- Utilising a person-centred approach
- Assisting the individual to meet their physical needs
- Working on improving cognitive ability including memory
- Reduce disorientation
- Being empathetic to the emotional context of memory loss and confusion
- Positively modify challenging behaviour

Assessments
- Risk
- History
- Symptoms
- Social functioning
- Quality of life
- Evaluation

Assessment skills
- Interview
- Observe
- Measure

Positive risk management
- Collaborative action planning and decision-making
- Thoughtful consideration of potential benefits and harms when deciding on actions
- Consider protective factors
- Ensuring that the risk management plan is fully communicated

Building a therapeutic relationship
- Using the right words
- Knowing when to be silent
- Using the right verbal and non-verbal responses
- Being an active listener and genuinely interested
- Accepting the person and being caring and compassionate

Communication underpinned by the 6Cs

Tree labels:
Bipolar affective disorder
Anxiety
Eating disorders
Depression
Learning disabilities and mental health
Personality disorders
Functional disorders in older adults
Dementia
Acute confusional states
Children and adolescent mental health
Children and adolescent mental health
Schizophrenia
Mental health law
Drug and alcohol misuse
Recovery
Psychological interventions
Medication and ECT
Classification
Physical wellbeing
Risk
Assessment
Lifelong learning
Reflection
Utilising research
Decision-making
Managing people
Time management
Leadership
Organising care
Medicines management
Documentation
Clinical observations
Elimination
Infection prevention and control
Nutrition and fluid management
Values-based practice
Managing clinical risk
Building therapeutic relationships
Care, compassion and communication

Scenario

Alex is seventy five years old and was diagnosed with dementia five years ago. He lived at home with his wife Ruth who has recently died; currently he lives with his daughter and her family. Alex has become increasingly aggressive and restless since moving in with his daughter's family and they are all struggling to cope with this behaviour. Recently Alex was found wandering the streets looking for his wife and claiming that people who he did not know had kidnapped him. His family had reported him missing but when he was found by the police he refused to go back home. He did agree to go into hospital and on this basis was admitted to a 'dementia' ward for further assessment. The student nurse with support from their mentor has been asked to assess Alex.

The practice tree in action

The assessment and care planning process can appear to be formulaic particularly when using an assessment tool. Obviously this process is more complex than this and involves skills and knowledge which is not always evident especially when being demonstrated by a skilled practitioner. The example above highlights some of the skills and knowledge that the student mental nurse will accrue as they journey towards being an effective practitioner. This example is not exhaustive and as a service user's condition changes then more factors may come into play which required additional skills and knowledge.

When considering the example above it is important to note that the assessment and planning process is not just about gathering information, communication and building an effective therapeutic relationship are key parts of this process, especially where a service user is in distress and feeling vulnerable. The assessment and planning process requires the nurse to have a specific set of skills and knowledge. They need to have the right skills such as knowing how to use open and probing questions; they also have to be competent in the use of specific assessment tools. In addition they have to be able to plan effectively, have a good understanding of dementia, and they would also be required to know which mental health nursing interventions should be delivered and why.

See 'Key Learning Points' in Chapters 1, 2, 11, 12, 13 & 23; and the companion website for further details.

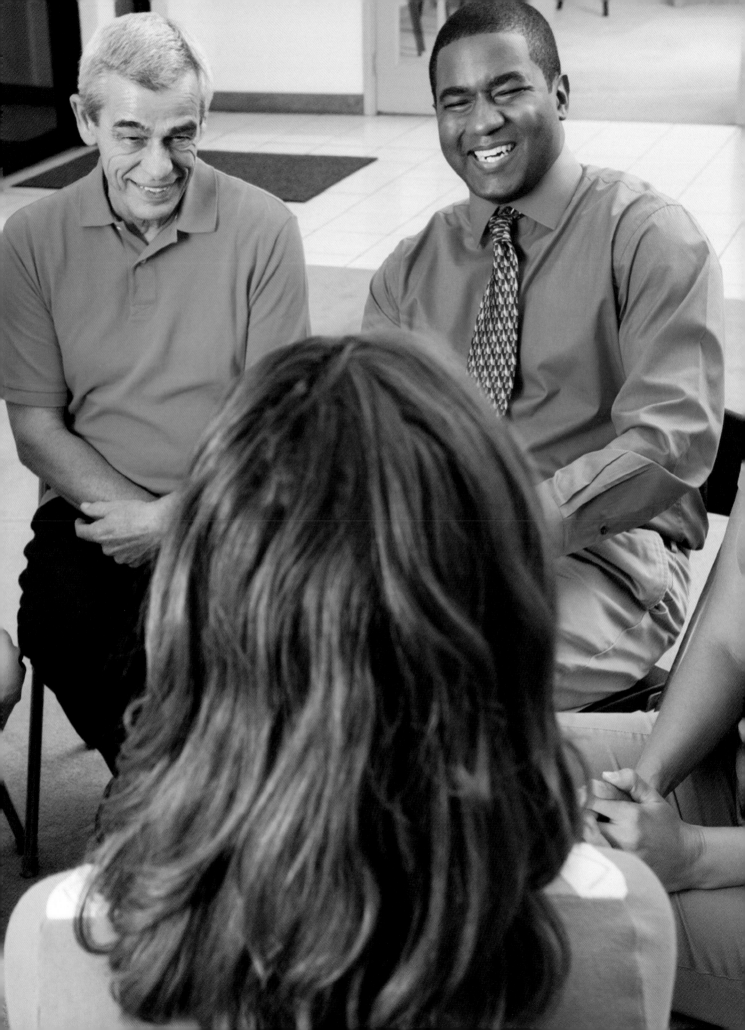

Essential skills

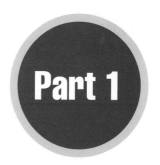

Part 1

Chapters

1 Care, compassion and communication 2
2 Building therapeutic relationships 4
3 Values-based practice 6
4 Managing clinical risk 8
5 Infection prevention and control 10
6 Nutrition and fluid management 12
7 Elimination 14
8 Clinical observations 16
9 Documentation 18
10 Medicines management 20

Don't forget to visit the companion website for this book www.ataglanceseries.com/nursing/mentalhealth to do some practice MCQs and case studies on these topics.

Care, compassion and communication

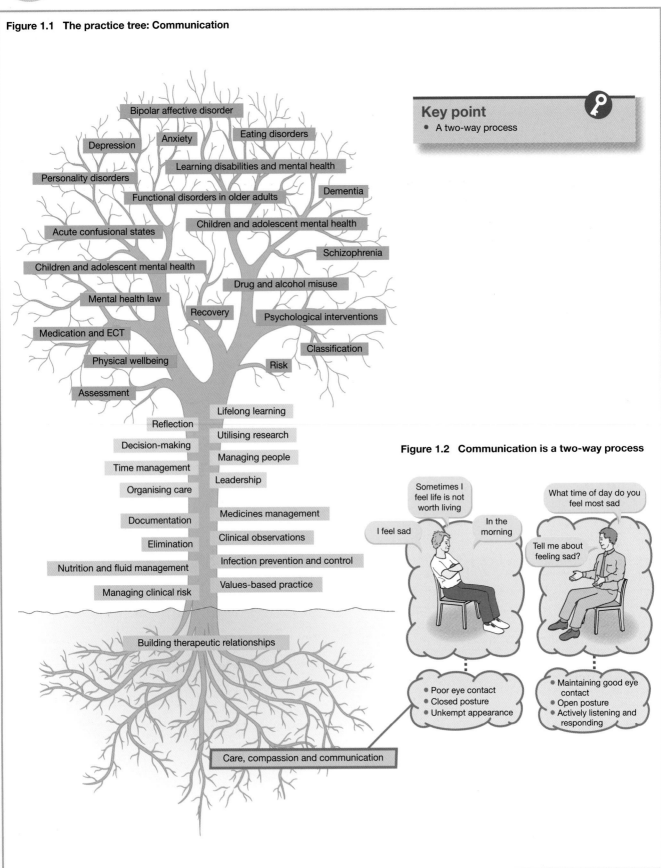

Figure 1.1 The practice tree: Communication

Key point
- A two-way process

Figure 1.2 Communication is a two-way process

Introduction

A mental health nurse is expected to demonstrate compassion when delivering care as well as being an effective communicator. Unlike most healthcare relationships the therapeutic relationship in mental health care is both the medium for treatment as well as in most cases the main treatment. Being an effective communicator gives the mental health nurse a platform from which to deliver a range of psychological interventions tailored to meet the specific needs of the mental health service user. Moreover, it is pivotal in the establishment and continuation of a therapeutic relationship that also manages risk, is recovery focused and has positive outcomes.

Professional competencies

Mental health nurses are required to:
- Have excellent communication, interpersonal and therapeutic skills.
- Be skilled in working in partnership with service users and carers.
- Engage in person-centred care that is compassionate and empowering.
- Preserve dignity, be anti-discriminatory and practise within the law considering such issues as confidentiality and consent.

The context

It is important to recognise that the more effective the communication skills of a mental health nurse, the more effective he or she will be in delivering care. Communication should be seen as a two-way process (Figure 1.2) in which information is shared between the service user and the mental health nurse; other people or agencies may also be part of this process. At times sharing information can be disrupted or blocked and this may be due to a number of factors. In these situations the responsibility lies with the mental health nurse as the competent practitioner, firstly to understand why this has happened and secondly to develop strategies to overcome any identified communication difficulties.

Types of communication

Communication can be broken down into verbal communication and non-verbal communication. Verbal communication can be seen to contain three key elements:
- The spoken word – vocals.
- The way the spoken word is expressed – paralanguage.
- The way the spoken word is perceived by the other person – meta-communication.

The majority of our communication is conveyed through non-verbal communication or body language, such as:
- facial expressions;
- eye contact;
- gestures
- posture;
- head movements;
- personal space;
- touch;
- appearance.

During the communication process the mental health nurse needs to be aware of their own body language and its impact upon the other person. They also need to be able to understand the potential messages that the other person's body language is conveying. Is the service user angry? are they sad? do they look confused? The mental health nurse will at times adapt their body language; if a service user is angry the mental health nurse will adopt a non-threatening but assertive posture.

Listening and responding

An important part of the communication process is that the nurse actively listens to what the service user is saying and then responds appropriately. The mental health nurse as an active listener must concentrate on what the service user is saying; this means that they must also control any potential distractions, giving the service user time and space to talk. The mental health nurse demonstrates that they are listening by responding in a way that is appropriate to what is being said. This can be achieved through the mental health nurse nodding their head – a non-verbal sign that they are listening; also the mental health nurse can summarise what the service user has said and then check or clarify with the service user that their understanding of what has been said is correct. A key part of understanding is based on the mental health nurse being skilled in asking open questions – "tell me about feeling sad" – and also being able to ask probing questions – "what time of day do you feel most sad?"

The 6 Cs

People with mental health needs can sometimes be highly vulnerable; it is essential in this situation that the mental health nurse shows empathy through a genuine understanding of the service user's experiences. This understanding should be based on the effective use of their communication skills but also through demonstrating such values and behaviours as:
- care;
- compassion;
- competence;
- communication;
- courage;
- commitment.

Further reading

Bowers, L. (2010) How expert nurses communicate with acutely psychotic patients. *Mental Health Practice* **13**(7): 24–26.

Department of Health (2013) Patients First and Foremost: The Initial Government Response to the Report of The Mid Staffordshire NHS Foundation Trust Public inquiry. London: Department of Health.

Hargie, O. (2006) *The Handbook of Communication Skills.* Hove: Routledge.

2 Building therapeutic relationships

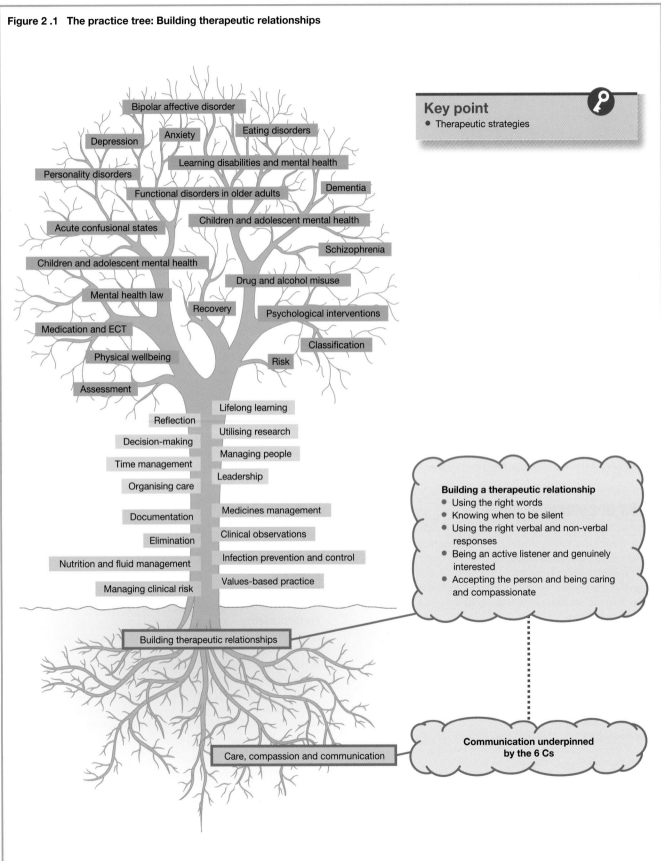

Figure 2 .1   The practice tree: Building therapeutic relationships

Bipolar affective disorder

Anxiety

Eating disorders

Depression

Learning disabilities and mental health

Personality disorders

Functional disorders in older adults

Dementia

Acute confusional states

Children and adolescent mental health

Children and adolescent mental health

Schizophrenia

Mental health law

Drug and alcohol misuse

Recovery

Medication and ECT

Psychological interventions

Physical wellbeing

Classification

Risk

Assessment

Lifelong learning

Reflection

Utilising research

Decision-making

Managing people

Time management

Leadership

Organising care

Documentation

Medicines management

Elimination

Clinical observations

Nutrition and fluid management

Infection prevention and control

Managing clinical risk

Values-based practice

Building therapeutic relationships

Care, compassion and communication

Key point
- Therapeutic strategies

Building a therapeutic relationship
- Using the right words
- Knowing when to be silent
- Using the right verbal and non-verbal responses
- Being an active listener and genuinely interested
- Accepting the person and being caring and compassionate

Communication underpinned by the 6 Cs

Mental Health Nursing at a Glance, First Edition. Grahame Smith. © 2015 John Wiley & Sons, Ltd. Published 2015 by John Wiley & Sons, Ltd.
Companion website: www.ataglanceseries.com/nursing/mentalhealth

Introduction

Therapeutic relationships in mental health nursing should be evidence-based, especially when delivering psychological interventions, and they should also respect the narrative of the service user. On this basis mental health nurses are required to build a therapeutic relationship that acknowledges the service user's diversity and at the same time delivers positive therapeutic outcomes. The therapeutic use of self is crucial within the process of developing meaningful and positive therapeutic relationships. It is also important to note that the use of self in a recovery-based relationship needs to be underpinned by the mental health nurse's commitment to partnership working.

Professional competencies

Mental health nurses are required to:
- Build safe therapeutic relationships that are partnership focused, person centred and non-discriminatory.
- Use relationship-building skills work with mental health service users, which includes being able to facilitate therapeutic groups.
- Use their personal qualities, experiences and interpersonal skills to build recovery-focused relationships.
- Be self-aware and know when to use self-disclosure while maintaining professional boundaries.
- Recognise mental distress and be able to respond using therapeutic principles that are underpinned by evidence-based practice.

The context

The therapeutic relationship is of central importance in the delivery of safe and effective mental health nursing interventions. These interventions where possible should be evidenced-based and they should also take into account the service user's narrative. At times it can become quite easy for the mental health nurse to reconstruct the service user's own experience of mental distress. This can happen, for example, when using an assessment tool that only captures the information the mental health nurse needs but does not capture the service user's entire story. Having different viewpoints can create conflict within the relationship unless the mental health nurse takes a collaborative approach. In addition the therapeutic relationship within the mental health field has a "risk element" where at times risk containment and risk minimisation shape the relationship. The impact is that although the therapeutic relationship is intended to be collaborative and person-centred, this intention can depend on the level of risk. Even so the nurse should always look to build therapeutic relationships that are based on true partnership working and at the same time value both the service user and their experiences – a person-centred philosophy.

The therapeutic self

Mental health nurses use a range of strategies in the process of building a therapeutic relationship (Figure 2.1). These strategies include:
- Selecting the right words to use.
- Knowing when to talk and when to be silent.
- Using the right verbal and non-verbal responses.
- Adapting non-verbal communication to suit the situation.

To use these strategies the mental health nurse needs to be self-aware. He or she needs to be aware of the impact their self has upon others, they need to be aware of their own thoughts and feelings, and they also need to be able to use this knowledge in a positive way when working with service users.

Empathy

It is essential within the therapeutic relationship that the mental health nurse is empathetic. This means that they have to be able to identify with the service user's experiences through being:
- an active listener;
- genuinely interested;
- accepting of the person;
- caring and compassionate.

Professional boundaries

Taking an empathetic approach gives the nurse the opportunity to be more thoughtful about the interventions they deliver, but also on occasion the nurse may self-disclose. As a therapeutic skill self-disclosure can be a way of fostering collaboration. When using self-disclosure the mental health nurse must remember that as a nursing professional there are professional boundaries that they must adhere to, with their conduct being governed by a professional code of conduct.

Reflection

To build therapeutic relationships that have positive outcomes the mental health nurse needs to be able to balance being person-centred and collaborative against the demands of being a clinical risk manager. To do this the mental health nurse has to be able to engage in reflection, which is a professional requirement as well as an important component of making effective clinical decisions and judgements. Reflection is a structured and critical process that requires the nurse to re-examine their practice experiences and focus on changing their practice for the better.

Further reading

Bracken, P. & Thomas, P. (2005) *Postpsychiatry: Mental Health in a Postmodern World*. Oxford: Oxford University Press.

Knott, D. (2012) From communication skills to psychological interventions. In: Smith, G. (ed.), *Psychological Interventions in Mental Health Nursing*. Maidenhead: Open University Press, pp. 24–26

Rigby, P. & Alexander, J. (2008) Building positive therapeutic relationships. In: Dooher, J. (ed.) *Fundamental Aspects of Mental Health Nursing*. London: Quay Books, pp. 103–16.

3 Values-based practice

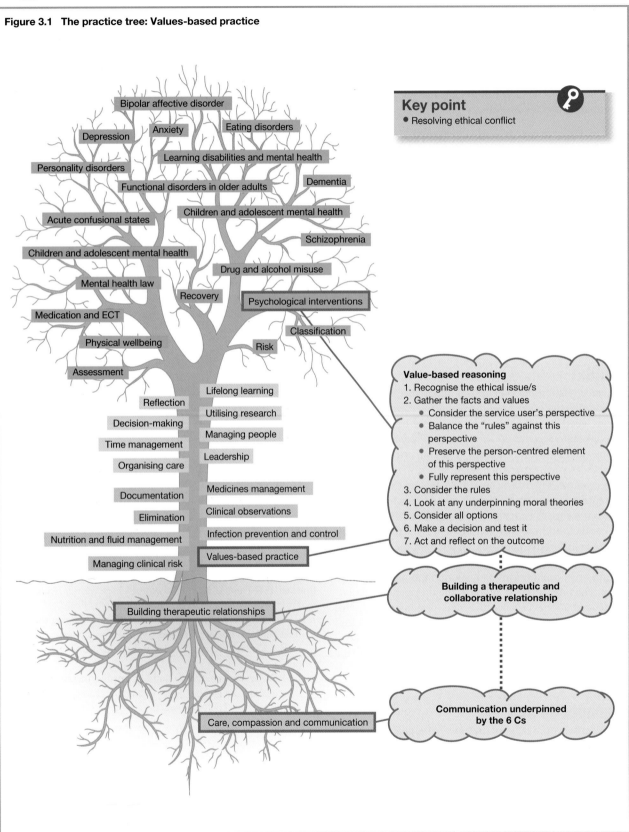

Figure 3.1   The practice tree: Values-based practice

Key point
- Resolving ethical conflict

Tree branches (labels):
- Bipolar affective disorder
- Anxiety
- Eating disorders
- Depression
- Learning disabilities and mental health
- Personality disorders
- Functional disorders in older adults
- Dementia
- Acute confusional states
- Children and adolescent mental health
- Schizophrenia
- Children and adolescent mental health
- Drug and alcohol misuse
- Mental health law
- Recovery
- Psychological interventions
- Medication and ECT
- Classification
- Physical wellbeing
- Risk
- Assessment
- Lifelong learning
- Reflection
- Utilising research
- Decision-making
- Managing people
- Time management
- Leadership
- Organising care
- Documentation
- Medicines management
- Elimination
- Clinical observations
- Nutrition and fluid management
- Infection prevention and control
- Values-based practice
- Managing clinical risk

Tree roots:
- Building therapeutic relationships
- Care, compassion and communication

Value-based reasoning
1. Recognise the ethical issue/s
2. Gather the facts and values
   - Consider the service user's perspective
   - Balance the "rules" against this perspective
   - Preserve the person-centred element of this perspective
   - Fully represent this perspective
3. Consider the rules
4. Look at any underpinning moral theories
5. Consider all options
6. Make a decision and test it
7. Act and reflect on the outcome

Building a therapeutic and collaborative relationship

Communication underpinned by the 6 Cs

Introduction

Mental health nurses are required to practice ethically; knowing how to act ethically is based on being able to utilise the relevant ethical theories, understand the relevant professional rules, and also having the skills to ethically reason. The added dimension for mental health nurses is that during the process of ethically reasoning they have also to take into account the value-laden nature of mental health practice.

Professional competencies

Mental health nurses are required to:
• Be able to understand the importance of values and beliefs and how they impact upon the communication process.
• Work within recognised professional, ethical and legal frameworks.
• Ensure that decisions about care are shared and in a way that values the meaning of a service user's experiences.
• Recognise and address ethical and legal challenges that arise within the therapeutic relationship.

The context

The mental health nurse is professionally expected to act ethically. To do this the mental health nurse must know "how to act ethically" and they must also be able to justify their actions. This need to act ethically is also contextualised by the controlling element of mental health nursing practice where the mental health nurse may in some cases have the power to restrict a service user's freedoms. By having this power to restrict freedoms there is potential for ethical conflict; for example, a mental health nurse may justify this power on the basis that they are keeping the service user safe, whereas the service user may see this power in more negative light, as an abuse of power. Where this conflict arises and different values are at play within the therapeutic relationship then this conflict needs to be managed in way that is collaborative and recovery-focused.

Ethical theory

Generally ethical theories that influence mental health nursing practice are normative ethical theories that focus on what actions are right, what ought to be done, what motives are good and what characteristics are virtuous:
• Consequentialism, also known as utilitarianism, is outcome focused; for the mental health nurse to be ethical their actions would need to produce the greatest balance of good over bad.
• Deontology, or Kantianism, is concerned with duty; the ethical mental health nurse without exception must always do their ethical/professional duty.
• Virtue ethics is based on the character of a person; a virtuous mental health nurse will acquire and utilise virtuous traits such as honesty, trustworthiness, cooperativeness and humility.

• Principlism is using principles in ethical decision-making, such as: do no harm (non-maleficence); act to benefit others (beneficence); respect a person's autonomy; and treat people fairly (justice).

Code of conduct

The Nursing and Midwifery Council as a professional body requires mental health nurses to follow a professional code, which is based on four ethical statements:
• Make the care of people your first concern, treating them as individuals and respecting their dignity.
• Work with others to protect and promote health and wellbeing of those in your care, their families and carers, and the wider community.
• Provide a high standard of practice and care at all times.
• Be open and honest, act with integrity and uphold the reputation of the profession.

Ethical reasoning

The code of conduct like ethical theories should underpin the mental health nurse's ethical reasoning endeavours; using an ethical framework can further assist this process:
1 Recognise the ethical issue/s.
2 Gather the facts and values.
3 Consider the rules.
4 Look at any underpinning moral theories.
5 Consider all options.
6 Make a decision and test it.
7 Act and reflect on the outcome.

Values-based practice

When gathering "facts" the mental health nurse also needs to gather "values". Values-based practice is a process that focuses on dealing with conflicting values rather than just focusing on the ethically right outcomes. This process requires the mental health nurse to work with values in a way that resolves ethical conflict (Figure 3.1) and then moves the therapeutic relationship forwards:
• Consider the service user's perspective.
• Balance the "rules" against this perspective.
• Preserve the person-centred element of this perspective.
• Fully represent this perspective in the decision-making process.

Further reading

Department of Health (2006) From Values to Action: The Chief Nursing Officer's Review of Mental Health Nursing. London: Department of Health.

Smith, G. (2012) Psychological interventions within an ethical context. In: Smith, G. (ed.), Psychological Interventions in Mental Health Nursing. Maidenhead: Open University Press, pp. 143–54.

Woodbridge, K. & Fulford, K.W.M. (2004) Whose Values? A Workbook for Values-based Practice in Mental Health Care. London: Sainsbury Centre for Mental Health.

4 Managing clinical risk

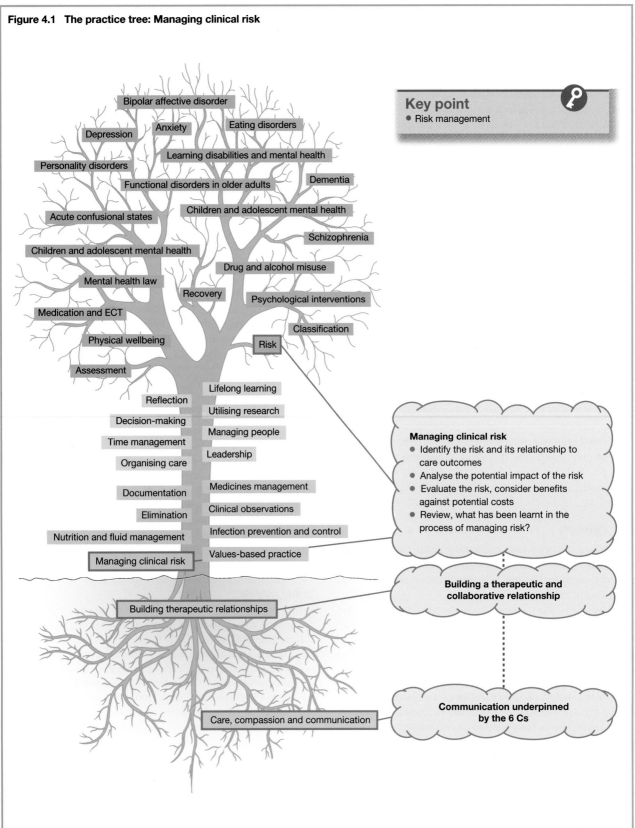

Figure 4.1 The practice tree: Managing clinical risk

Key point
- Risk management

Managing clinical risk
- Identify the risk and its relationship to care outcomes
- Analyse the potential impact of the risk
- Evaluate the risk, consider benefits against potential costs
- Review, what has been learnt in the process of managing risk?

Building a therapeutic and collaborative relationship

Communication underpinned by the 6 Cs

(Tree labels:)
Bipolar affective disorder
Anxiety
Eating disorders
Depression
Learning disabilities and mental health
Personality disorders
Dementia
Functional disorders in older adults
Acute confusional states
Children and adolescent mental health
Children and adolescent mental health
Schizophrenia
Drug and alcohol misuse
Mental health law
Recovery
Psychological interventions
Medication and ECT
Classification
Physical wellbeing
Risk
Assessment
Lifelong learning
Reflection
Utilising research
Decision-making
Managing people
Time management
Leadership
Organising care
Documentation
Medicines management
Elimination
Clinical observations
Nutrition and fluid management
Infection prevention and control
Managing clinical risk
Values-based practice
Building therapeutic relationships
Care, compassion and communication

Mental Health Nursing at a Glance, First Edition. Grahame Smith. © 2015 John Wiley & Sons, Ltd. Published 2015 by John Wiley & Sons, Ltd.
Companion website: www.ataglanceseries.com/nursing/mentalhealth

Introduction

Mental health nurses are required to manage clinical risk, though there is a tendency to focus on a service user's risk to self and others rather than seeing risk as a wider issue (also see Chapter 12). Clinical risk management in a wider context focuses on keeping users of services safe. To do this you have to be able to identify potential hazards and risks. Within mental health care the nurse also has to take into consideration that managing clinical risk should be a process that is partnership focused.

Competencies

Mental health nurses are required to:
• Recognise risk.
• Manage risk in a way that is person-centred and recovery-focused.
• Be aware of the potential risks of the care they deliver.
• Report concerns promptly, and change care where required to maintain safety.
• Manage risk both independently and as part of a team approach.

The context

Risk relates to the threat or likelihood that an adverse action or event will occur. Therefore, clinical risk management is concerned with the development of strategies that prevent such an action or event from occurring, or if prevention is not possible the focus would be on minimising harm/s. Hazards and risks can include events that involve staff and carers as well as service users. These events would include deliberate self-harm and violence to others, to slips and falls, and also administrative errors that may have a negative impact upon care.

Risk

Risks are adverse incidents that are waiting to happen, whereas a hazard is something that has the potential to cause harm, such as a slippery floor that has not been dealt with. Clinical risk refers to risk within a care delivery context. Mental health nurses tend to use the language of risk in way that includes hazards; it is also used to refer to the potential of something going wrong when delivering care. Incidents could include:
• medication incidents;
• consent and capacity incidents;
• control and restraint incidents;
• breaches in confidentiality;
• accidents to staff, service users and visitors;
• environmental incidents such as flood and fire.

This use of the term in this narrow way tends to focus on worrying about clinical errors rather than managing risk holistically. On this basis risk needs to be framed in terms of a managed and holistic process.

Risk management

Risk management (Figure 4.1) is a systematic process of identifying and then managing risk through preventing, eliminating or minimising the identified risk:
• Identify the risk and its relationship to care outcomes.
• Analyse the potential impact of the risk.
• Evaluate the risk – consider benefits against potential costs.
• Review – what has been learned in the process of managing risk?

In terms of nursing practice the mental health nurse needs to have systems in place that focus on keeping themselves safe and the people they work with. Part of the risk management process also requires the mental health nurse to learn from their experiences of encountering adverse incidents, and as a future action change their behaviour to reduce the potential of the event occurring again. Learning from incidents both at an individual level and at an organisational level requires the mental health nurse to be effective in how they communicate and also document the issues that have arisen.

Risk and organisational culture

Risk management is not just about preventing risk; for an organisation to grow it must at times take risks but these risks need to be identified and managed. For example, on the basis of promising evidence a NHS Trust may want to introduce a new psychological intervention into the care of people living with dementia. Before introducing this intervention the Trust would need to identify the risks and the benefits, and if they decide to go ahead they would need to develop an action plan that manages those identified risks.

Clinical governance

Risk management is a component of clinical governance, which is a process or system where healthcare organisations are required to keep improving the quality of the services they provide. To do this organisations are required to safeguard high standards of care through promoting a working environment in which excellent care will grow. For clinical governance to work effectively there must be:
• Clinical governance policies and procedures that also include the management of risk.
• Clear lines of responsibility and accountability.
• Quality improvement systems in place.
• Education and training plans.
• Procedures to identify and manage concerns about the quality of care.

Further reading

National Patient Safety Agency (NPSA) (2007) *Healthcare Risk Assessment Made Easy*. London: NPSA.

NHS Quality Improvement Scotland (2010) *Vital Systems, Supporting Healthcare Improvement in Scotland – Person-centred Safe and Effective Care: Clinical Governance and Risk Management a National Overview*. Edinburgh: NHS QIS.

Ottewill, M., Renshaw, M. & Carmody, J. (2006) Using patient and staff stories to improve risk management. *Nursing Times* **102**(8): 34.

5 Infection prevention and control

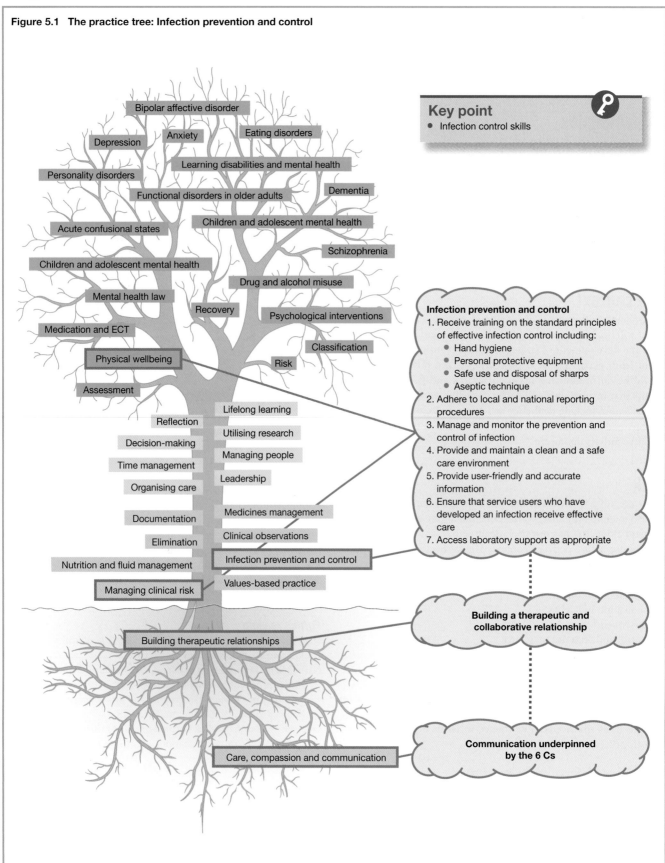

Figure 5.1 The practice tree: Infection prevention and control

Bipolar affective disorder

Anxiety

Eating disorders

Depression

Learning disabilities and mental health

Personality disorders

Functional disorders in older adults

Dementia

Acute confusional states

Children and adolescent mental health

Children and adolescent mental health

Schizophrenia

Mental health law

Drug and alcohol misuse

Recovery

Medication and ECT

Psychological interventions

Classification

Physical wellbeing

Risk

Assessment

Lifelong learning

Reflection

Utilising research

Decision-making

Managing people

Time management

Leadership

Organising care

Documentation

Medicines management

Elimination

Clinical observations

Nutrition and fluid management

Infection prevention and control

Managing clinical risk

Values-based practice

Building therapeutic relationships

Care, compassion and communication

Key point
- Infection control skills

Infection prevention and control
1. Receive training on the standard principles of effective infection control including:
   - Hand hygiene
   - Personal protective equipment
   - Safe use and disposal of sharps
   - Aseptic technique
2. Adhere to local and national reporting procedures
3. Manage and monitor the prevention and control of infection
4. Provide and maintain a clean and a safe care environment
5. Provide user-friendly and accurate information
6. Ensure that service users who have developed an infection receive effective care
7. Access laboratory support as appropriate

Building a therapeutic and collaborative relationship

Communication underpinned by the 6 Cs

Mental Health Nursing at a Glance, First Edition. Grahame Smith. © 2015 John Wiley & Sons, Ltd. Published 2015 by John Wiley & Sons, Ltd.
Companion website: www.ataglanceseries.com/nursing/mentalhealth

Introduction

Mental health nurses deliver different clinical interventions; the majority of these inventions are psychosocial. Yet it is easy to forget that mental health nurses are at times required to provide physical health care such as clinical observations and wound care amongst many other interventions. When delivering these interventions it is important that the mental health nurse follows principles that focus on preventing and controlling infections.

Competencies

Mental health nurses are required to:
• Adhere to local and national policies on the prevention and control of infection.
• Apply agreed infection control and prevention practices in all environments.
• Provide effective nursing care in the case of infectious diseases including the use of isolation techniques.
• Act to reduce risk when handling sharps, contaminated linen and clothing and when dealing with body fluid spillages.

The context

Infection control and prevention aims to have a zero tolerance of infection; mental health nurses have a key role to play in achieving this aim. It is also important to remember that when delivering physical health care there is always risk, such as cross-infection; in this context the mental health nurse will need to manage these risks. Part of managing these risks is to implement effective infection control procedures; the other part requires the mental health nurse to frame their practice through the risk management process (see Chapter 4).

Physical health interventions

Mental health nurses deliver a number of physical health interventions that require the nurse to think about infection control and prevention. The following is an illustrative list of some of those interventions:
• pulse;
• blood pressure;
• temperature;
• wound care;
• administering injections;
• collecting a sputum sample;
• peak flow;
• urinalysis;
• testing blood glucose;
• first aid;
• basic life support.

Spreading of infections

Micro-organisms can be spread in different ways:
• aerosol;
• droplet;
• faecal–oral;
• person-to-person, most often by contaminated hands.
• indirect contact such as through food, water and inanimate objects;
• body fluids;
• insects and parasites.

Infection control practices

There is a national drive to ensure that infection control practices are consistent whatever the environment. This is important for mental health nurses as they can practise within a wide variety of health and social care settings. There is an emphasis on maintaining standards through training, and establishing systems that ensure consistent and reliable practice; also there is a focus on clinical leaders acting as infection control role models. To maintain consistency generally mental health nurses need to:
• Receive training on the standard principles of effective infection control and prevention.
• Adhere to local and national reporting procedures for infections.
• Manage and monitor the prevention and control of infection using a robust risk assessment process.
• Provide and maintain a clean and a safe care environment.
• Provide user-friendly and accurate information on infections and infection control to service users and carers.
• Ensure that service users who develop an infection receive care that aims to reduce the risk of passing on the infection to others.
• Access laboratory support as appropriate.

Infection control skills

Effective infection prevention and control (Figure 5.1) ensures that people who access health and social care services receive safe care. On this basis mental health nurses should be trained in:
• hand hygiene;
• personal protective equipment;
• safe use and disposal of sharps;
• aseptic technique.

Further reading

Hughes, J., Blackman, H., McDonald, E., Hull, S. & Fitzpatrick, B. (2011) Involving service users in infection control practice. *Nursing Times* **107**: 25

National Institute for Health and Clinical Excellence (NICE) (2012) Infection: Prevention and control of healthcare-associated infections in primary and community care – Clinical Guideline 39. London: NICE.

Royal College of Nursing (RCN) (2012) *Essential Practice for Infection Prevention and Control: Guidance for Nursing Staff.* London: RCN.

6 Nutrition and fluid management

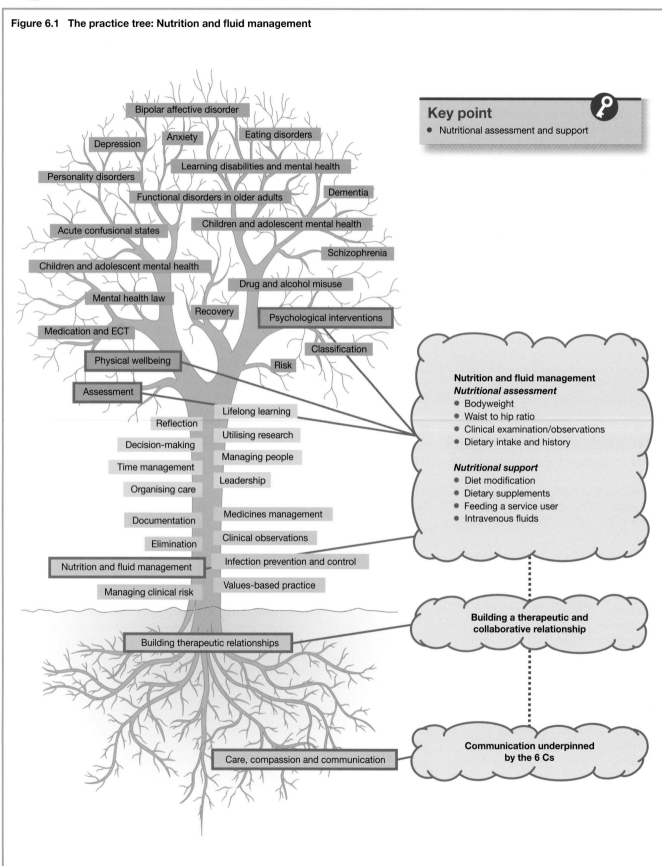

Figure 6.1   The practice tree: Nutrition and fluid management

Bipolar affective disorder

Anxiety

Depression

Eating disorders

Personality disorders

Learning disabilities and mental health

Functional disorders in older adults

Dementia

Acute confusional states

Children and adolescent mental health

Children and adolescent mental health

Schizophrenia

Mental health law

Drug and alcohol misuse

Recovery

Medication and ECT

Psychological interventions

Physical wellbeing

Classification

Risk

Assessment

Lifelong learning

Reflection

Utilising research

Decision-making

Managing people

Time management

Leadership

Organising care

Documentation

Medicines management

Elimination

Clinical observations

Nutrition and fluid management

Infection prevention and control

Managing clinical risk

Values-based practice

Building therapeutic relationships

Care, compassion and communication

Key point

- Nutritional assessment and support

Nutrition and fluid management
Nutritional assessment
- Bodyweight
- Waist to hip ratio
- Clinical examination/observations
- Dietary intake and history

Nutritional support
- Diet modification
- Dietary supplements
- Feeding a service user
- Intravenous fluids

Building a therapeutic and collaborative relationship

Communication underpinned by the 6 Cs

Mental Health Nursing at a Glance, First Edition. Grahame Smith. © 2015 John Wiley & Sons, Ltd. Published 2015 by John Wiley & Sons, Ltd.
Companion website: www.ataglanceseries.com/nursing/mentalhealth

Introduction

Nutritional health is the foundation for good physical and mental wellbeing. It is generally recognised that mental health service users can struggle with poor nutrition and a lack of physical activity. This may relate to service users' social circumstances such as living in more deprived areas or difficulty in gaining employment; it may also relate to the side-effects of psychiatric medication. Whatever the causes, it is known that mental health service users have an increased risk of mortality and physical illness. On this basis mental health nurses play a key role in promoting good nutritional health within their client group (Figure 6.1).

Competencies

Mental health nurses are required to:
• Assess and monitor diet and fluid status and where required formulate effective plans of care.
• Support service users in choosing and maintaining a healthy nutritional and fluid intake.
• Ensure that service users who are unable to take food and fluids by mouth receive adequate fluid and nutrition to meet their needs.

The context

Maintaining a balanced diet, which includes drinking enough water, is essential for good health and wellbeing. When someone is physically unwell, depending on the condition and the circumstances, this can negatively impact upon their ability to maintain a balanced diet, and if the person then becomes malnourished this can adversely affect their recovery. Being malnourished can impair a person's immune response, delay wound healing and also increase the risk of mortality and developing other physical problems and illnesses. To maintain a balanced diet a person needs, in the right amounts:
• carbohydrates;
• proteins;
• fats;
• vitamins;
• minerals.

A specific issue within the field of mental health is the issue of weight gain. Service users treated with antipsychotic medication are more likely to be clinically obese than the general population. This in turn can increase an individual's chances of developing diabetes and coronary heart disease. Taking this into consideration once an individual commences antipsychotic treatment it is important that their weight is monitored regularly and action is taken where there are concerns about weight gain.

Assessing nutrition and fluid intake

Managing nutrition requires the mental health nurse to assess a service user's nutritional status. This assessment should be part of a continuous process where information can be compared over a period of time. Especially in the case of weight gain where actual weight gain is identified over a specific time period, this information can then be compared against nutritional intake and activity data. The type of information collected should include:
• Bodyweight – Body Mass Index.
• Waist-to-hip ratio.
• Clinical examination/observations as appropriate – physical appearance, oedema, mobility, mood, wound healing.
• Dietary intake, over a 24-hour period.
• Diet history, such as food frequency, food habits, meal pattern, portion size and any eating difficulties.

Nutrition support

Within the in-patient setting nutritional support may range from providing a specific diet to assisting service users to eat and drink. The support provided will depend on the service users' identified needs and their level of dependence. Interventions may include:
• Diet modification such as providing smaller and more regular meals, or increasing or reducing a specific food group.
• Dietary supplements such as specific vitamins and/or minerals.
• Feeding a service user – where possible self-feeding should be encouraged throughout and supported.
• Enteral tube feeding – providing a specific feed through a tube directly into the service user's gastrointestinal tract.
• Intravenous fluids – these may be given where a service user is dehydrated.

When providing nutritional support it is important to recognise that a number of factors may impact upon a service user's ability to eat and drink independently. These can include:
• Difficulties in chewing and swallowing.
• Weakness or stiffness or paralysis affecting the arms, hands and/or fingers.
• Mobility problems that adversely affect a service user's ability to position themselves while eating.

Health promotion

Where a service user is independent then nutritional support may take the form of promoting a good diet, which could include referring the service user to a dietician. It is important to note that changing your diet is a lifestyle change. On this basis the mental health nurse may be required to undertake motivational work to support the service user in their efforts to make a sustainable change to their eating habits.

Further reading

Aneurin Bevan Health Board (2010) Guidelines for the treatment of under nutrition in the community including advice on oral nutritional supplement (sip feed) prescribing. Pontypool: Aneurin Bevan Health Board.

Johnstone, C. & Farley, A. (2006) Nurses' role in nutritional assessment and screening – Part one of a two-part series. *Nursing Times* **102**(49): 28.

National Institute for Health and Clinical Excellence (2006) Nutrition support in adults: Oral nutrition support, enteral tube feeding and parenteral nutrition – Clinical Guideline 32. London: NICE.

7 Elimination

Figure 7.1 The practice tree: Elimination

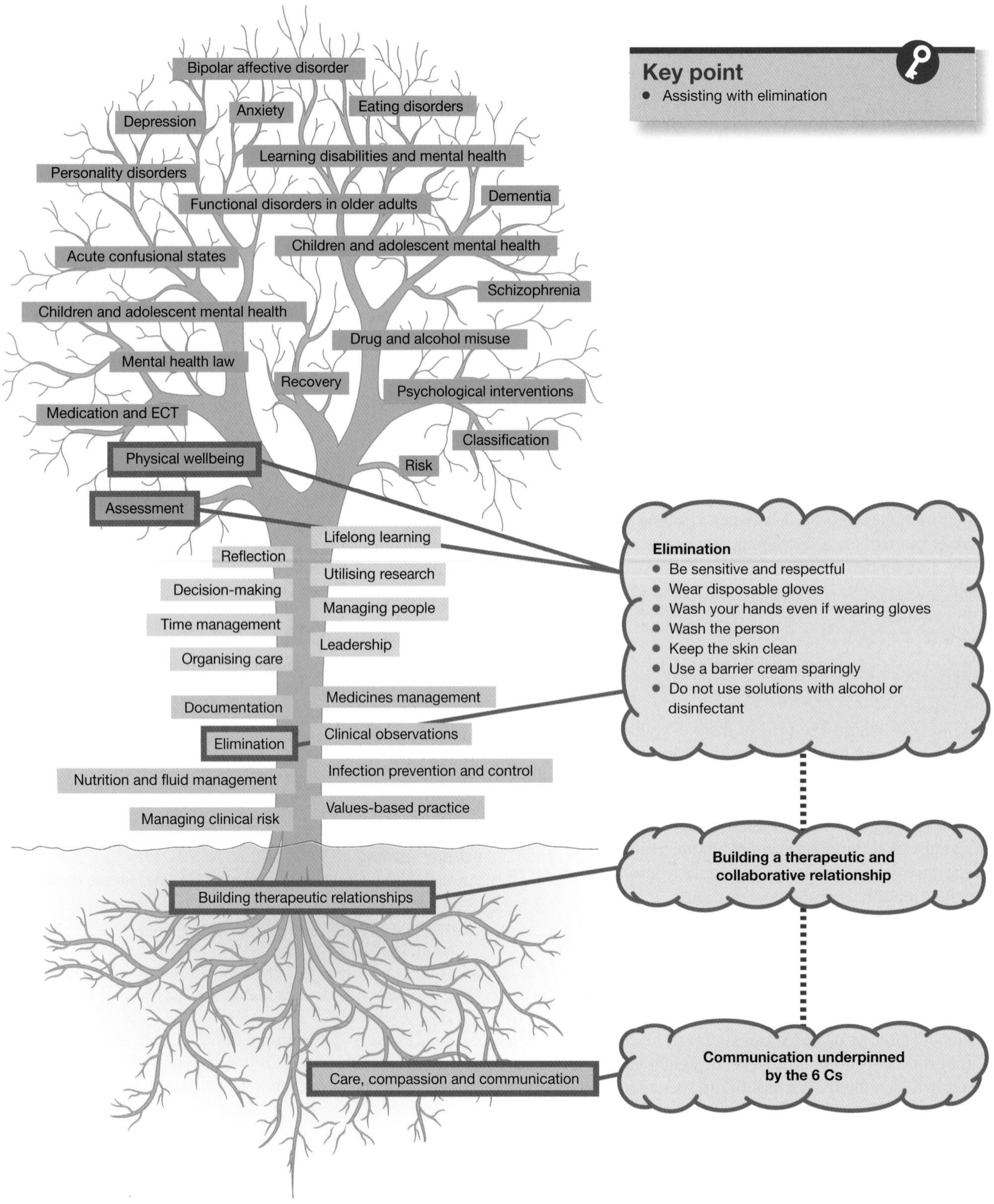
Bipolar affective disorder
Depression
Anxiety
Eating disorders
Learning disabilities and mental health
Personality disorders
Functional disorders in older adults
Dementia
Children and adolescent mental health
Acute confusional states
Schizophrenia
Children and adolescent mental health
Drug and alcohol misuse
Mental health law
Recovery
Psychological interventions
Medication and ECT
Classification
Physical wellbeing
Risk
Assessment
Lifelong learning
Reflection
Utilising research
Decision-making
Managing people
Time management
Leadership
Organising care
Documentation
Medicines management
Elimination
Clinical observations
Nutrition and fluid management
Infection prevention and control
Managing clinical risk
Values-based practice
Building therapeutic relationships
Care, compassion and communication
Elimination
Be sensitive and respectful
Wear disposable gloves
Wash your hands even if wearing gloves
Wash the person
Keep the skin clean
Use a barrier cream sparingly
Do not use solutions with alcohol or disinfectant
Building a therapeutic and collaborative relationship
Communication underpinned by the 6 Cs

Key point

- Assisting with elimination

Companion website: www.ataglanceseries.com/nursing/mentalhealth

Introduction

Supporting mental health service users to meet their own physical needs can be a sensitive issue, especially when dealing with bowel and bladder care. The majority of mental health service users will be able to independently meet their own "elimination" needs. In this case the mental health nurse's role will focus on providing support and advice where personal hygiene issues arise. When a service user is unable to independently meet their elimination needs the mental health nurse should offer effective care that respects and maintains dignity.

Competencies

Mental health nurses are required to:
• Provide safe, person-centred care for service users who are unable to meet their own physical needs.
• Act with dignity and respect to ensure that service users who are unable to meet their own physical needs feel empowered.
• Deliver care that meets service users' essential needs such as bowel and bladder care.
• Work collaboratively to ensure an adequate fluid intake and output.

The context

Assisting service users to manage their elimination needs requires not only a sensitive approach but also partnership working between the mental health nurse and the service user. For this assistance to be effective the mental health user has to obtain consent; where a service user is unable to provide consent their rights need to be protected. The type of assistance provided may range from prompting and reminding an individual to go to the toilet, to providing equipment such as commodes or bedpans. If physical assistance is required – whether this is with or without equipment – a manual handling assessment needs to be undertaken. It also has to be recognised that although most individuals have a bowel and bladder routine this routine can be quite specific to the individual and their circumstances.

Elimination assessment

Elimination is the excretion of urine and faecal matter from the body. When assessing service users' bowel and bladder routines it is important to note the level of support they require and whether they have any concerns. Other types of information you might collect are the:
• Frequency, volume, consistency and colour.
• Presence of blood, mucus, undigested food or offensive smell.
• Report of pain and/or discomfort.
• Urinalysis.

Incontinence

Incontinence is an inability to control the function of the bladder or bowel; this can be due to a dysfunction and/or underlying health problem. In most cases incontinence can be managed effectively through a continence management and treatment regime. Types of incontinence include:
• Stress incontinence – a leakage of urine that usually happens during physical activity.
• Urge incontinence – an uncontrollable urge to pass urine and at times an individual may find it difficult to make it to the toilet in time.
• Overflow incontinence – where an individual uncontrollably passes small amounts of urine during the day and night.
• Reflex incontinence – usually a complete leakage of urine without the individual having a feeling of needing to go to the toilet or having control.
• Constipation – where the stools become difficult to pass.
• Faecal incontinence – where there is a loss of control of the bowels.

Assisting with elimination

It is important to recognise that within a hospital environment a service user's incontinence problems may simply reflect their inability to reach the toilet in time. this could be due to mobility difficulties or not knowing where the toilet is located. Some ward environments manage these issues by good signage and by having two-hourly rounds. In terms of rounds this is where nurses routinely engage with the service users, focusing on personal care including bladder and bowel care. This does not mean that a service user's specific elimination needs are not dealt with outside these times. While undertaking bowel and bladder care (Figure 7.1) the nurse must remember to:
• Wear disposable gloves.
• Wash hands even if wearing gloves.
• Wash the person.
• Keep the skin clean.
• Use a barrier cream sparingly and preferably a cream that has a pH near to that of normal skin.
• Not use solutions with alcohol or disinfectant.

Within a home environment the mental health nurse should work with other agencies to ensure that a service user's independence is maintained; this may include adapting the environment so that a service user has easy and safe access to toileting facilities.

Further reading

National Institute for Health and Clinical Excellence (2007) *Faecal incontinence: the management of faecal incontinence in adults – clinical guideline 49.* London: NICE.

Royal College of Nursing (RCN) (2006) *Improving Continence Care for Patients: The Role of the Nurse.* London: RCN.

Royal College of Nursing (2008) *Catheter Care: RCN Guidance for Nurses.* London: RCN.

8 Clinical observations

Figure 8.1 The practice tree: Clinical observations

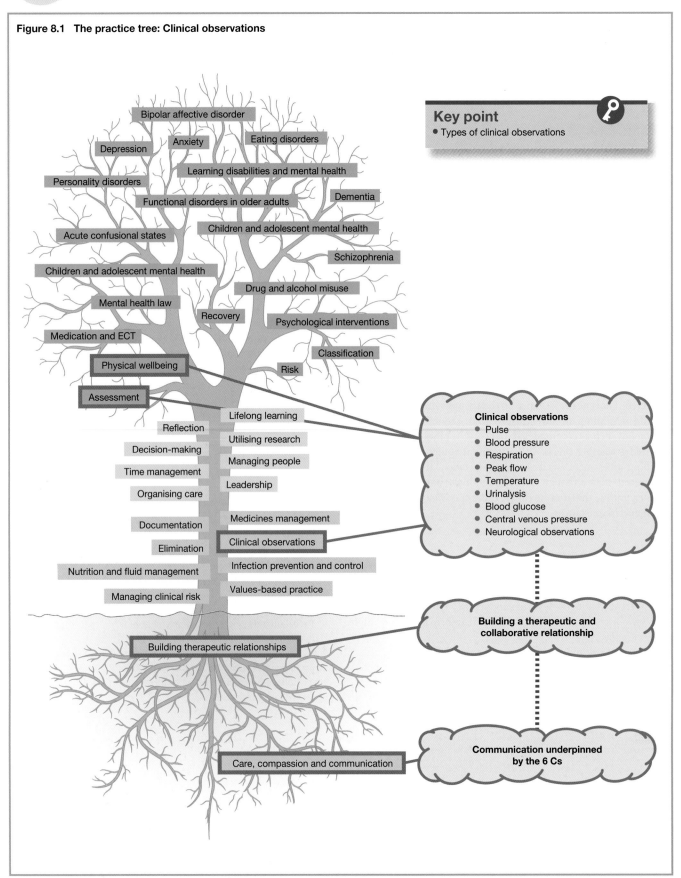

Bipolar affective disorder
Anxiety
Eating disorders
Depression
Learning disabilities and mental health
Personality disorders
Functional disorders in older adults
Dementia
Acute confusional states
Children and adolescent mental health
Schizophrenia
Children and adolescent mental health
Drug and alcohol misuse
Mental health law
Recovery
Psychological interventions
Medication and ECT
Classification
Physical wellbeing
Risk
Assessment

Lifelong learning
Reflection
Utilising research
Decision-making
Managing people
Time management
Leadership
Organising care
Documentation
Medicines management
Elimination
Clinical observations
Nutrition and fluid management
Infection prevention and control
Managing clinical risk
Values-based practice

Building therapeutic relationships

Care, compassion and communication

Key point
- Types of clinical observations

Clinical observations
- Pulse
- Blood pressure
- Respiration
- Peak flow
- Temperature
- Urinalysis
- Blood glucose
- Central venous pressure
- Neurological observations

Building a therapeutic and collaborative relationship

Communication underpinned by the 6 Cs

Mental Health Nursing at a Glance, First Edition. Grahame Smith. © 2015 John Wiley & Sons, Ltd. Published 2015 by John Wiley & Sons, Ltd.
Companion website: www.ataglanceseries.com/nursing/mentalhealth

Introduction

A key part of the mental health nurse's role is to develop a comprehensive and personalised plan of care; this plan of care needs to consider a service user's physical health needs. To ensure that a service user's physical needs are systematically assessed the mental health nurse has to undertake a number of clinical observations.

Competencies

Mental health nurses are required to:
• Collect and interpret routine data related to the care planning process.
• Be able to measure and record a service user's weight, height, temperature, pulse, respiration and blood pressure.
• Respond appropriately where a service user's vital signs are outside the normal range or where there is a sudden deterioration in a service user's vital signs.
• Carry out and interpret routine diagnostic tests such as a urinalysis.

The context

Undertaking clinical observations is an important but sometimes forgotten part of the mental health nurse's role, especially when you consider that mental health service users will have higher rates of physical health needs than the general population. In the long term, for clinical observation data to be meaningful, they need to be integrated with information obtained from other sources such as clinical examination and medical history data. In the short term, clinical observation or vital sign data can assist in the process of determining whether you are dealing with a physical emergency (Figure 8.1). Clinical observations include:
• pulse;
• blood pressure;
• respiration;
• peak flow;
• temperature;
• urinalysis;
• blood glucose;
• central venous pressure;
• neurological observations.
Clinical observations that are sometimes called vital signs historically consist of temperature, pulse, respiratory rate and blood pressure. Besides these vital signs mental health nurses also need to be familiar with peak flow, urinalysis and blood glucose. See Appendix for more information on some of the above procedures.

Pulse

Measuring the pulse gives an indication of how the heart is functioning; counting the pulse, or beats per minute, is equivalent to measuring heart rate. A 'normal' pulse rate for a healthy adult is between 60 and 100 beats per minute. The pulse can be felt in any place that allows an artery to be compressed against a bone, such as the neck, wrist, knee, inside of the elbow and near the ankle joint. The pulse is usually taken at the wrist – the radial site; besides the rate, the rhythm and amplitude (pulse strength) are also noted.

Respiratory rate

The role of the respiratory system is to ensure that the body has enough oxygen and that carbon dioxide is removed; this respiratory process consists of:
• Ventilation – movement of air in and out of the lungs.
• External respiration – gas exchange.
• Transport – movement of respiratory gases.
• Internal respiration – delivery of oxygen and uptake of carbon dioxide.
Generally a respiratory assessment consists of assessing the:
• Airway – checking for obstructions.
• Breathing – rate, rhythm and depth.
• Skin colour – looking for cyanosis, a blue tone to the skin.
• Use of accessory muscles – such as breathing through flared nostrils or pursed lips.
• General condition – level of consciousness.

Blood pressure

Blood pressure is a measure of the force of blood or pressure against the vessel walls such as the brachial artery in the upper arm, the usual site for measuring blood pressure. Blood pressure as a value is expressed as systolic pressure over diastolic pressure; systolic pressure reflects the peak pressure of the left ventricle in the heart, and diastolic pressure reflects aortic pressure at its lowest. Normal blood pressure which is measured in millimetres of mercury (mmHg) can range from 110 to 140 mmHg for systolic pressure, and from 70 to 80 mmHg for diastolic pressure. Where an individual's sustained blood pressure is measured as being greater than 140/90 mmHg this can be defined as hypertension; if they have a systolic reading less than 100 mmHg this can be defined as hypotension.

Temperature

Temperature can be too high or too low. A normal body temperature range is 36.0 to 37.2 °C; below 35.0 °C it is called hypothermia and above 37.5 °C it is called pyrexia. Temperature readings can be taken by non-digital thermometers or digital thermometers, usually at these sites: mouth, forehead, ear canal and under the arm.

Further reading

Boulanger, C. & Toghill, M. (2009) How to measure and record vital signs to ensure detection of deteriorating patients. *Nursing Times* **105**(47): 10–12.

Castledine, G. (2006) The importance of measuring and recording vital signs correctly. *British Journal of Nursing* **15**(5): 285.

Watson, D. (2006) The impact of accurate patient assessment on quality of care. *Nursing Times* **102**(6): 34–7.

9 Documentation

Figure 9.1 The practice tree: Documentation

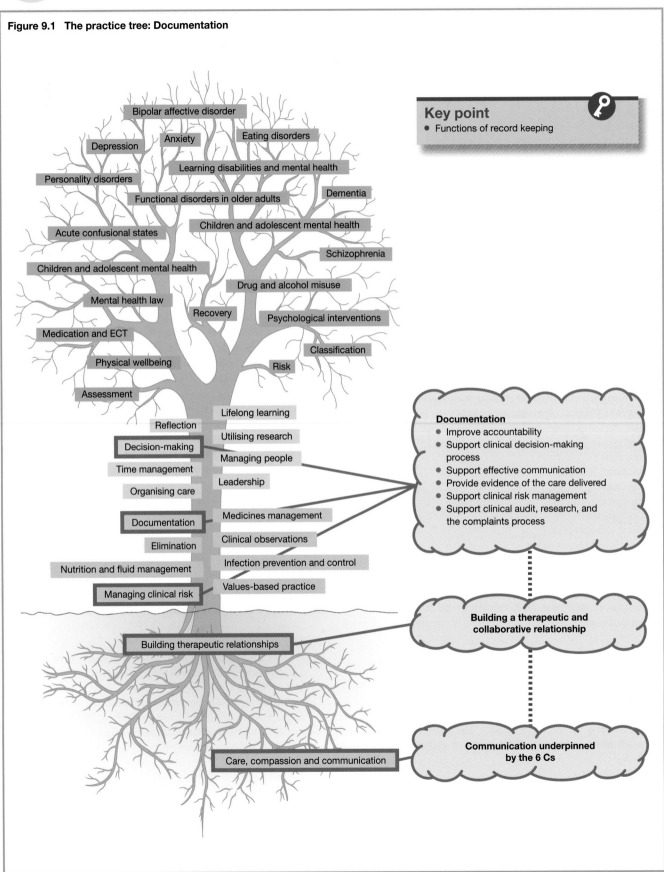

Key point
- Functions of record keeping

Documentation
- Improve accountability
- Support clinical decision-making process
- Support effective communication
- Provide evidence of the care delivered
- Support clinical risk management
- Support clinical audit, research, and the complaints process

Building a therapeutic and collaborative relationship

Communication underpinned by the 6 Cs

Tree labels:
- Bipolar affective disorder
- Anxiety
- Eating disorders
- Depression
- Learning disabilities and mental health
- Personality disorders
- Functional disorders in older adults
- Dementia
- Acute confusional states
- Children and adolescent mental health
- Children and adolescent mental health
- Schizophrenia
- Mental health law
- Drug and alcohol misuse
- Recovery
- Psychological interventions
- Medication and ECT
- Classification
- Physical wellbeing
- Risk
- Assessment
- Lifelong learning
- Reflection
- Utilising research
- Decision-making
- Managing people
- Time management
- Leadership
- Organising care
- Documentation
- Medicines management
- Elimination
- Clinical observations
- Nutrition and fluid management
- Infection prevention and control
- Managing clinical risk
- Values-based practice
- Building therapeutic relationships
- Care, compassion and communication

Mental Health Nursing at a Glance, First Edition. Grahame Smith. © 2015 John Wiley & Sons, Ltd. Published 2015 by John Wiley & Sons, Ltd.
Companion website: www.ataglanceseries.com/nursing/mentalhealth

Introduction

Recording the planning and delivering of care is an important and an essential part of mental health nursing practice. These records should provide a clear and accurate record of the care delivery process; they should also adhere to the guidance on record keeping of the Nursing and Midwifery Council (NMC). When recording care the mental health nurse will need to find a balance between their professional view of a given situation and the service user's view; they will then need to find an agreed viewpoint. To ensure that there is a balance when recording care information this process should be person-centred and collaborative.

Professional competencies

Mental health nurses are required to:
• Ensure they maintain records that are based on the best available evidence and that these records are accurate, clear and complete, whatever the format.
• Fully participate in the care-planning process, which includes completing relevant documentation and also evaluating the outcome of any planned interventions.
• Document care that fully identifies the service user's needs including taking appropriate action where required.
• Manage record keeping in a way that adheres to the relevant professional and legal frameworks.

The context

Professionally record keeping is viewed as "essential to the provision of safe and effective care". Records are also part of the communication process where better communication means that there is a better quality of care delivered. For example, if a service user's condition is clearly and accurately recorded other members of the care team over time should be able to detect whether there have been any changes to the service user's condition and then act accordingly. Certainly this is important where there are constant changes to the personnel delivering care, such as in the case of shift-pattern working. As mental health nurses work in different settings, within and also outside the NHS, then records may be kept in different formats from "paper" records to records that are only available in an "electronic" format. Whatever the format the principles of good record keeping remain the same as do the core professional values of individuality and partnership working. Types of records include:
• handwritten clinical notes;
• emails and text messages;
• clinical letters;
• X-rays, laboratory reports and printouts;
• incident reports and statements;
• photographs and videos.

The function of documentation

Documentation is used in many contexts (Figure 9.1) and is used for a number of purposes such as:
• Improving accountability.
• Presenting and supporting the clinical decision-making process.
• Supporting effective communication.
• Providing documentary evidence of the care delivered.
• Supporting the clinical risk management process.
• Supporting clinical audit, research and the complaints process.

Documentation standards

A mental health nurse's clinical record keeping needs to adhere to the NMC's guidance/standards. The following is a summarised list of those standards; it is recommended that the guidance is read in full:
• Handwriting should be legible and all entries should be fully signed, with the date and time.
• The entry should be accurate, factual and the meaning clear with no unnecessary jargon.
• Professional judgement should be used to decide what should be recorded.
• Information related to a service user's care should be fully recorded.
• Records should not be altered and/or destroyed without the relevant authorisation.
• Any authorised alteration must be fully signed with the original entry record still clearly readable or auditable.
• Ensure that the record-keeping process adheres to the relevant professional and legal frameworks as well as national and local policies.
• Service users and carers should where appropriate be involved in the record-keeping process.
• Information that is not clinically relevant should not be kept.
• Service users need to be aware that their clinical records may be seen by other people or agencies involved in their care.

Improving record keeping

It is essential that mental health nurses adhere to the professional guidance on record keeping. But they also need to reflect on how they can continually improve their practice. When engaging in this process of reflection it might be useful to consider:
• Does your entry provide accurate evidence of the standard of care delivered?
• Is it person-centred?

Further reading

Nursing and Midwifery Council (NMC) (2011) *Guidance on Professional Conduct: For Nursing and Midwifery Students.* London: NMC

Royal College of Nursing (2012) *Delegating Record Keeping and Countersigning Records: Guidance for Nursing Staff.* London: RCN.

Stevens, S. & Pickering, D. (2010) Keeping good nursing records: a guide. *Community Eye Health* **23**(74): 44–45.

10 Medicines management

Figure 10.1 The practice tree: Medicines management

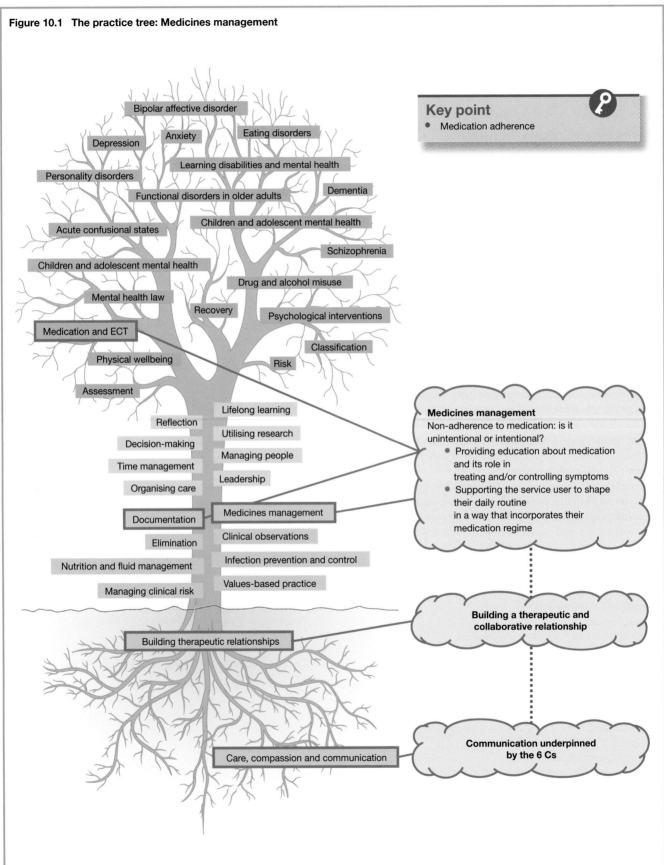

Mental Health Nursing at a Glance, First Edition. Grahame Smith. © 2015 John Wiley & Sons, Ltd. Published 2015 by John Wiley & Sons, Ltd.
Companion website: www.ataglanceseries.com/nursing/mentalhealth

Introduction

Medicines management is an important component of mental health nursing practice especially where medication is utilised as a front-line treatment. Medication management is not just concerned with the administration of medication but has a broader role to play. As an example, medication can support the service user's journey to recovery but only if medicines management is viewed as part and parcel of the therapeutic relationship. The value of this approach is that the service user is viewed as a collaborative partner in a process that aims to enable them to make autonomous decisions about their prescribed medication.

Professional competencies

Mental health nurses are required to:
• Ensure that managing medicines is built on safe and effective practice that is underpinned by a commitment to work in partnership.
• Administer medicines and keep and maintain records that relate to medicine management in accordance with the relevant professional standards.
• Ensure that their medicine management practice adheres to the relevant ethical-legal frameworks and also to the relevant national and local policy guidelines.

The context

Administering medication is an important part of medicines management. To ensure that mental health nurses safely and effectively administer medication they need to consider the issue of adherence. This issue is not unique to the mental health field; medication adherence (Figure 10.1) is a major challenge for all healthcare professionals. If a person does not take their medication as prescribed it can impact adversely on their recovery as well as their health and wellbeing. Not adhering to a medication regime can be:
• Unintentional – such as when the person forgets to take their medication.
• Intentional – where the person decides not to take their medication.
To enhance adherence the mental health nurse should consider:
• Providing education about medication and its role in treating and/or controlling the symptoms of the identified health condition.
• Supporting the service user to shape their daily routine in a way that incorporates their medication regime; they should also be encouraged to talk about the drawbacks and the benefits of taking medication.

Medication management standards

In terms of nursing practice, when managing medicines mental health nurses should adhere to the NMC's guidance/standards. The following is a summarised list of those standards; it is recommended that the guidance is read in full:
• Methods – medication must only be supplied and administered via a patient specific direction (PSD) or patient medicines administration chart.
• Checking – any direction to administer a medicinal product must be checked.
• Prescription medicines – in exceptional circumstances and with certain conditions a nurse may label from stock and supply a clinically appropriate medicine.
• Storage – all medicinal products are to be stored in accordance with their UK licence.
• Transportation – nurses may transport medication to service users in certain cases and under certain conditions.
• Administration – the nurse must be certain of the identity of the service user, and that they are not allergic to the medicine. The nurse must know the therapeutic uses of the medicine to be administered, its normal dosage, side-effects, precautions and contraindications. The nurse must check the expiry date of the medicine and that the prescription is clearly written and unambiguous; the method of administration, route and timing must also be considered.
• Assessment – the nurse is responsible for the initial and continued assessment of patients who are self-administering.
• Remote prescription or direction to administer – in exceptional circumstances and under certain conditions the use of information technology (such as fax, text message or email) may be used.
• Titration – where medication has been prescribed within a range of doses, it is acceptable for nurses to titrate doses.
• Preparing medication in advance – a nurse must not prepare substances for injection in advance.
• Nursing students – students must never administer or supply medicinal products without direct supervision.
• Management of adverse effects – if a nurse makes an error they must take action to prevent any potential harm to the service user and report the incident as soon as possible.

Further reading

Barber, P. (2013) *Medicine Management for Nurses: Case Book.* Maidenhead: Open University Press.

Barber, P. & Robertson, D. (2012) *Essentials of Pharmacology for Nurses*, 2nd edn. Maidenhead: Open University Press.

British National Formulary (http://www.bnf.org/bnf/index.htm).

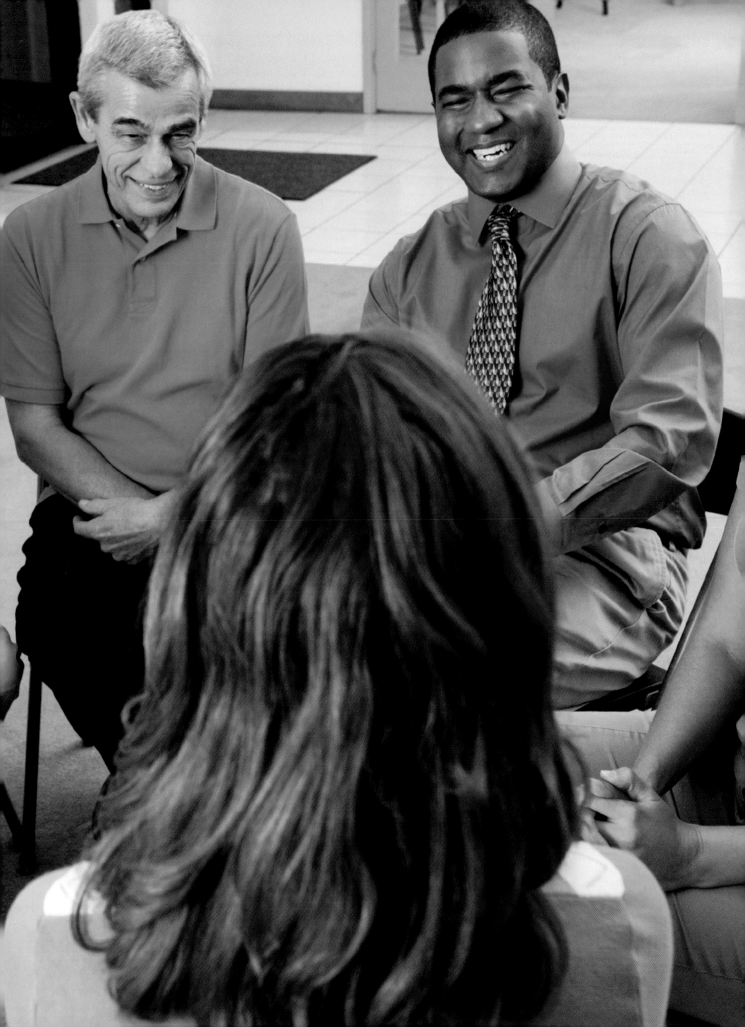

Nursing individuals with mental health needs

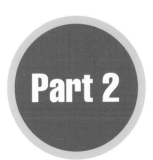

Part 2

Chapters

Don't forget to visit the companion website for this book www.ataglanceseries.com/nursing/mentalhealth to do some practice MCQs and case studies on these topics.

11 Assessment 24

12 Risk 26

13 Classification 28

14 Psychological interventions 31

15 Schizophrenia 34

16 Depression 36

17 Bipolar affective disorder 38

18 Anxiety 40

19 Eating disorders 42

20 Personality disorders 44

21 Learning disabilities and mental health 46

22 Functional disorders in older adults 48

23 Dementia 50

24 Acute confusional states 52

25 Drug and alcohol misuse 54

26 Children and adolescent mental health 56

27 Recovery 58

28 Physical wellbeing 60

29 Mental health law 62

30 Medication and ECT 66

11 Assessment

Figure 11.1   The practice tree: Assessment

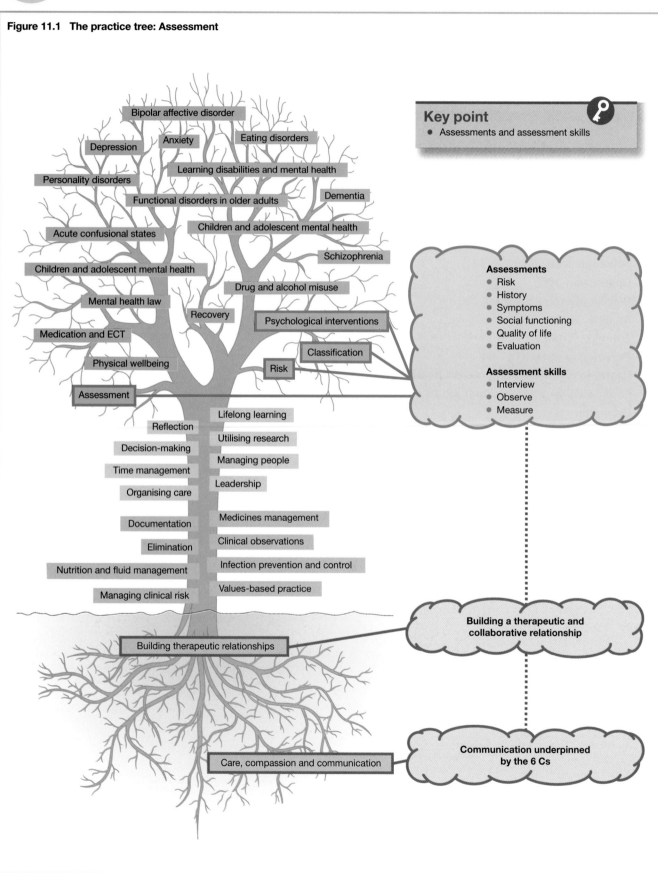

Key point
- Assessments and assessment skills

Assessments
- Risk
- History
- Symptoms
- Social functioning
- Quality of life
- Evaluation

Assessment skills
- Interview
- Observe
- Measure

Building a therapeutic and collaborative relationship

Communication underpinned by the 6 Cs

Tree labels:
Bipolar affective disorder
Anxiety
Eating disorders
Depression
Learning disabilities and mental health
Personality disorders
Functional disorders in older adults
Dementia
Acute confusional states
Children and adolescent mental health
Children and adolescent mental health
Schizophrenia
Drug and alcohol misuse
Mental health law
Recovery
Psychological interventions
Medication and ECT
Classification
Physical wellbeing
Risk
Assessment

Lifelong learning
Reflection
Utilising research
Decision-making
Managing people
Time management
Leadership
Organising care
Documentation
Medicines management
Elimination
Clinical observations
Nutrition and fluid management
Infection prevention and control
Managing clinical risk
Values-based practice

Building therapeutic relationships

Care, compassion and communication

Introduction

Assessment is a fundamental part of mental health nursing practice; it is about establishing an understanding of a service user's situation through a process of asking questions. This process is not a one-off; it should be an ongoing process, built on partnership working, which starts with a service user's admission to services and continues until they are discharged. It is worth noting that a service user's care journey may cut across a number of care settings so it is crucial that assessment information seamlessly follows the service user throughout this journey. Information gathered from the assessment process is the first step in planning and delivering care; therefore, to ensure that the care delivered is effective, the mental health nurse needs to collect the right information.

Professional competencies

Mental health nurses are required to:
- Undertake nursing assessments that are comprehensive, systematic and holistic.
- Utilise assessment information to plan, deliver and evaluate care.
- Throughout the assessment process work in partnership with the service user, their carers and their families, to negotiate goals and develop a personalised plan of care.

The context

Assessment can be broadly divided into two categories or methods:
- Formal assessment includes checklists, questionnaires, rating scales, tools and structured interviews.
- Informal assessment is where information is collected through less formal and planned methods such as day-to-day observations and interactions.

Both methods provide the nurse with valuable information and both should have equal weight, though formal assessment tends to be viewed as being more objective and value free. Sometimes this can lead to information gathered through formal assessment methods having more weight than informally gathered information. The strength of using both methods is that information can be triangulated in a way that captures the whole clinical picture rather than just part of the picture. On this basis assessment information should describe the service user's situation, both generally and specifically; it should also identify the degree to which any identified problem has and is impacting upon the service user's ability to function. To elicit this information the nurse would use:
- Open questions to scope the broad issues.
- More probing questions to identify the specific issues.
- Closed questions to confirm that the service user's understanding of the specific issues is correct.

Types of assessments

Mental health nursing assessments should be holistic, which means that through the assessment process the nurse will gather a wide range of information within the following areas:
- physical health and functioning;
- psychological functioning;
- social functioning;
- spiritual.

Dependent on the capabilities of the nurse they may use a variety of assessment tools to gather specific information about:
- risk;
- history;
- symptoms;
- social functioning;
- quality of life.

Assessment tools

Specific assessment tools used in mental health nursing include:
- Brief Psychiatric Scale;
- Beck Depression Inventory;
- Positive and Negative Syndrome Scale;
- Beliefs About Voices Questionnaire;
- Self-Esteem Scale;
- Health of the Nation Outcome Scales;
- Camberwell Assessment of Need;
- Social Functioning Scale;
- Quality of Life Scale;
- Patient Health Questionnaire.

Assessment skills

The development of the therapeutic relationship should drive the assessment process (Figure 11.1). As a process it should be person-centred, collaborative and underpinned by the use of effective communication skills such as questioning, active listening, clarifying and summarising. The mental health nurse is goal focused – what information do I need to collect and how? They may:
- Interview – ask questions about behaviours and symptoms.
- Observe – record what they see.
- Measure – rate the severity of behaviours and symptoms.

Ordinarily they would utilise all three strategies. It is also important to focus on what the service user can do rather than what they cannot do; this strengths approach underpins the recovery process.

Assessment and care delivery

Assessment information is used to inform the delivery of care. It assists the mental health nurse and service user in partnership to identify what the issues are and what needs to be addressed. The next step is to consider as a partnership "what are we trying to achieve?" and "what change would we like to take place and by when?" After this step the partnership would consider what interventions would be the most useful; also at this stage the relevant clinical guidelines would need to be taken into consideration. Finally, "did we achieve our goals, if not why not?"; "is there another approach we could consider?" Overall the process looks like this:
- assessment;
- care planning and goal setting;
- care delivery;
- evaluation.

Further reading

Curran, J. & Rogers, P. (2004) Acute psychiatric in-patient assessment. In: Harrison, M., Howard, D. & Mitchell, D. (eds), *Acute Mental Health Nursing: From Acute Concerns to the Capable Practitioner*. London: Sage, pp. 9–29.

Grant, A., Mills, J., Mulhern, R. & Short, N. (2004) The therapeutic alliance and case formulation. In: Grant, A., Mills, J., Mulhern, R. & Short, N. (2004) *Cognitive Behavioural Therapy in Mental Health Care*. London: Sage, pp. 7–22.

Smith, G. (2012) An introduction to psychological interventions. In: Smith, G. (ed.), *Psychological Interventions in Mental Health Nursing*. Maidenhead: Open University Press, pp. 1–10.

12 Risk

Figure 12.1 The practice tree: Risk

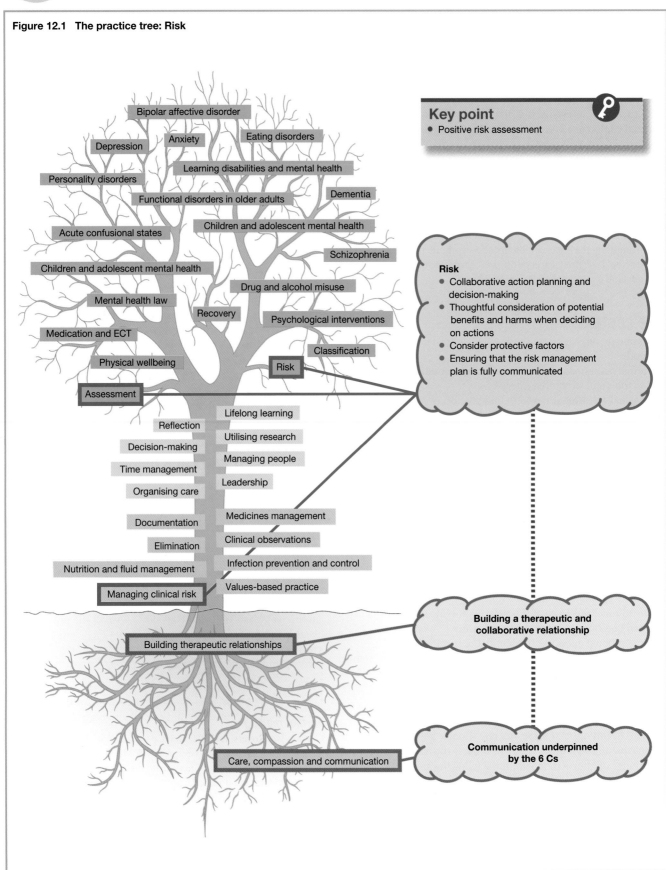

Key point
- Positive risk assessment

Bipolar affective disorder

Anxiety

Eating disorders

Depression

Learning disabilities and mental health

Personality disorders

Functional disorders in older adults

Dementia

Children and adolescent mental health

Acute confusional states

Children and adolescent mental health

Schizophrenia

Drug and alcohol misuse

Mental health law

Recovery

Psychological interventions

Medication and ECT

Classification

Physical wellbeing

Risk

Assessment

Lifelong learning

Reflection

Utilising research

Decision-making

Managing people

Time management

Leadership

Organising care

Documentation

Medicines management

Elimination

Clinical observations

Nutrition and fluid management

Infection prevention and control

Managing clinical risk

Values-based practice

Building therapeutic relationships

Care, compassion and communication

Risk
- Collaborative action planning and decision-making
- Thoughtful consideration of potential benefits and harms when deciding on actions
- Consider protective factors
- Ensuring that the risk management plan is fully communicated

Building a therapeutic and collaborative relationship

Communication underpinned by the 6 Cs

Mental Health Nursing at a Glance, First Edition. Grahame Smith. © 2015 John Wiley & Sons, Ltd. Published 2015 by John Wiley & Sons, Ltd.
Companion website: www.ataglanceseries.com/nursing/mentalhealth

Introduction

This chapter follows on from Chapter 4 in Part 1 on managing clinical risk. The focus of this chapter will be on managing risk within a specific context – where there is the potential that a mental health service user poses a risk to self and/or others. Risk management in this context still needs to be partnership focused; it also needs to be systematic. This process will be dynamic in nature as levels of risk can change quite quickly and at times it can be controlling, especially where risk is managed through the use of legally restricting an individual's freedoms.

Competencies

Mental health nurses are required to:
• Recognise and manage risk in a way that is person-centred, recovery-focused and protects vulnerable individuals.
• Manage risk in a way that empowers choices and promotes wellbeing.
• Work positively and proactively with individuals who are at risk, using evidence-based models of care that prevent, reduce and minimise risk.
• Manage risk both independently and as part of a team approach in a way that promotes effective communication, positive risk management and continuity of care across services.

The context

Managing risk within the context of mental health care relates to the threat or likelihood that harm to self and/or others will occur. To manage this potential risk the mental health nurse will undertake an assessment of risk; any risks identified will be documented and communicated appropriately to the multi-disciplinary team. The next stage is to systematically manage risk through the implementation of a risk management plan.

Risk assessment

Managing risk within the field of mental health has been influenced by a number of governmental initiatives and policies, one of these being the Care Programme Approach (CPA). On this basis when assessing risk the mental health nurse needs to consider:
• Type of risk – self-harm, neglect, to others and from others.
• How recent were the risk-related incidents? How severe is the risk and what is the level of intent?
• How frequent have the risk-related incidents been?
• When do they happen? Are there trigger factors? Does the individual use drugs and alcohol at the same time?
• What is the service user's understanding of the identified risks? What is their present mental state like and do they have capacity?

Type of risk assessments

Risk assessment approaches include:
• Unstructured risk assessment – where clinical risk information is accrued unsystematically.
• Actuarial risk assessment – where risk information is collected and processed through a number of statistically based categories using a risk assessment tool and a risk score is calculated.

• Structured risk assessment – where evidence-based research influences the types of risk information collected usually through the use of specific risk assessment tools. This information is then compared with the nurse's knowledge of the service user and the service user's own views.

In terms of best practice a structured approach is the best approach, though this is dependent on the skill of the nurse and the availability of suitable risk assessment tools.

Managing risk

Managing risk should be based on a positive risk management approach with a focus on collaboration and recovery (Figure 12.1) and especially when engaging in 'supportive observations' of service users at risk. The level of supportive observation is implemented as indicated by the level of identified risk:
• Level 1, or general observation, is the minimum level of observations for all in-patients.
• Level 2, or intermittent observation, is where the service user's location on the ward is checked every 15 to 30 minutes.
• Level 3 observation is where the service user is kept within sight at all times.
• Level 4 observation is where the service user is kept within arm's length of the observing nurse.

Using a positive and supportive approach prevents over-defensive practice and promotes therapeutic engagement. A positive approach would include:
• Actively listen to the service user's views.
• Collaborative action planning and decision-making.
• Thoughtful consideration of potential benefits and harms when deciding on actions.
• Implementing decisions that involve an element of risk where the benefits outweigh the risks.
• Ensuring that the risk management plan is fully communicated.

When managing risk it is useful to note that risks can be static or dynamic. Static risks are risk-related incidents that have happened (history) or factors such as age or employment that statistically indicate that an individual is at risk. Dynamic risks relate to factors that constantly influence risk such as an individual's mental state or their social circumstances. By taking into account the dynamic nature of risk and how these may change over time, the nurse can not only identify the present risk, but also consider the impact these dynamic factors have on the service user's level of risk at that point in time. These factors can also be protective especially in the case where a service user has:
• the skills and the psychological resources to cope;
• meaningful work;
• a social network that is supportive.;
• access to the right services.

Further reading
Care Programme Approach Association (CPAA) (2008) *The CPA and Care Standards Handbook*, 3rd edn. Chesterfield: CPAA.
Department of Health (2007) *Best Practice in Managing Risk: Principles and Evidence for Best Practice in the Assessment and Management of Risk to Self and Others in Mental Health Services*. London: Department of Health.
Department of Health (2010) *Nothing Ventured, Nothing Gained: Risk Guidance for People with Dementia*. London: Department of Health.

13 Classification

Figure 13.1 The practice tree: Mental health nursing interventions

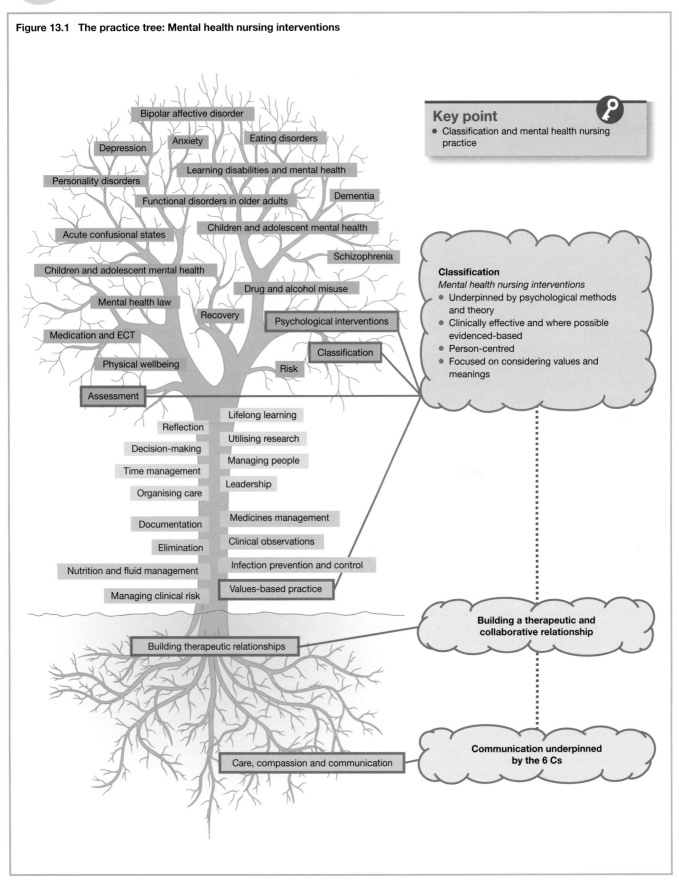

Key point
- Classification and mental health nursing practice

Classification
Mental health nursing interventions
- Underpinned by psychological methods and theory
- Clinically effective and where possible evidenced-based
- Person-centred
- Focused on considering values and meanings

Building a therapeutic and collaborative relationship

Communication underpinned by the 6 Cs

Tree labels:
- Bipolar affective disorder
- Anxiety
- Eating disorders
- Depression
- Learning disabilities and mental health
- Personality disorders
- Functional disorders in older adults
- Dementia
- Acute confusional states
- Children and adolescent mental health
- Children and adolescent mental health
- Schizophrenia
- Mental health law
- Drug and alcohol misuse
- Recovery
- Psychological interventions
- Medication and ECT
- Classification
- Physical wellbeing
- Risk
- Assessment
- Reflection
- Lifelong learning
- Decision-making
- Utilising research
- Time management
- Managing people
- Organising care
- Leadership
- Documentation
- Medicines management
- Elimination
- Clinical observations
- Nutrition and fluid management
- Infection prevention and control
- Managing clinical risk
- Values-based practice
- Building therapeutic relationships
- Care, compassion and communication

Mental Health Nursing at a Glance, First Edition. Grahame Smith. © 2015 John Wiley & Sons, Ltd. Published 2015 by John Wiley & Sons, Ltd.
Companion website: www.ataglanceseries.com/nursing/mentalhealth

Introduction

Psychiatrists conceptualise mental distress that is greater than the statistical norm as mental illness. This term is broken down into groupings or classifications, which include:
- organic disorders;
- psychotic disorders;
- mood disorders;
- anxiety disorders;
- personality disorders.

These disorders are further specified through a diagnostic process that is supported by internationally agreed frameworks or classification systems. It is important to acknowledge that psychiatric diagnoses do not fit as easily into the practice of the mental health nurse as they do for the psychiatrist. A fundamental problem with this approach for mental health nurses is that classifying or applying labels is not holistic enough to identify all the needs of mental health service users. Nonetheless, mental health nurses have to be able to understand and work with this approach as diagnosis and classification is a fundamental form of communication used throughout mental health care.

Competencies

Mental health nurses are required to:
- Recognise different forms of mental distress and respond effectively irrespective of the service user's age or setting.
- Understand the impact that an individual's mental distress can have upon their ability to function.
- Apply and value the use of evidence within their practice.
- Have an in-depth understanding of how mental disorders relate to the care and treatment of individuals with mental health needs.

The context

At the turn of the 20th century mental distress was starting to be described in the following terms:
- unconscious processes;
- thinking processes and behaviours;
- brain pathology;
- neurotransmitters.

As psychiatry became a specific medical discipline there was a greater interest in systematically describing mental distress as mental illness. The work of Emil Kraepelin (1856–1923) started to link symptoms to distinct syndromes or disorders, and the work of Karl Jaspers (1883–1969) started to formulate a common language of mental disorder based on describing signs and symptoms.

Classification

Classifying mental illnesses is viewed as providing a scientific basis on which the practice of psychiatry can be built upon. It also aims to provide a framework that improves:
- The diagnostic process – reliability and validity.
- Communication – common language.
- Treatment outcomes and clinical management.

Figure 13.2 Mental health nursing interventions

DSM-IV-TR (multiaxial and categorical)	ICD-10 (categorical)
Axis I	
Disorders usually first diagnosed in infancy, childhood, or adolescence	F80–89 Disorders of psychological development
	F90–98 Onset specific to childhood and adolescence
Delirium, dementia, and amnestic and other cognitive disorders	F00–09 Organic
Substance-related disorders	F10–19 Due to substance use
Psychotic disorders	F20–29 Psychotic disorders
Mood disorders	F30–39 Mood (affective) disorders
Anxiety disorders	F40–48 Neurotic, stress related and somatoform disorders
Somatoform disorders	
Factitous disorders	
Dissociative disorders	
Adjustment disorders	
Eating disorders	F50–59 Behavioural syndromes associated with physiological disturbances and physical factors
Sleep disorders	
Sexual and gender identity disorders	F60–69 Personality disorders, habit and impulse disorders, disorders of sexual preference and gender identity disorders
Impulse-control disorders	
Axis II	
Personality disorders	
Mental retardation	F70–79 Mental retardation
Axis III	
General medical conditions	
Axis IV	
Psychosocial and environmental problems	
Axis V	
Global assessment of functioning, on a scale from 100 (excellent functioning) to 0.	

There are two established frameworks for classifying mental disorders: the *International Classification of Diseases* (ICD; Chapter 5: Mental and Behavioural Disorders), and the *Diagnostic and Statistical Manual of Mental Disorders* (DSM). The ICD was established in 1993 and is now in its 10th edition; at the time of writing the 11th edition is planned for release in 2015. DSM was established in 1952, the fifth edition was released early 2013 and is currently in the process of being implemented; at the time of writing the fourth edition is still widely used (see Figure 13.2). Both frameworks are distinct but generally they complement each other.

Diagnosis

The diagnostic process is an assessment process where the focus is on collecting information, firstly to understand what the issues are and secondly to formulate a treatment plan. This process has two distinct parts:

* the psychiatric history and mental state examination;
* the formulation.

This process provides the psychiatrist with information related to the presenting problem, the history of this problem, and a description of the individual's behaviour and mental experiences at the time the assessment process is carried out. The formulation summarises what the issues are; it is at this stage that a diagnosis is usually applied, and based on the best evidence the treatment plan is then formulated.

Mental health nursing practice

Mental health nurses usually have the greatest amount of direct contact with mental health service users. This unique position should shape the care the mental health nurse delivers. The knowledge generated from being in this unique position must be used to complement the information gathered from the diagnostic process. Using a psychiatric diagnosis on its own provides only limited information as it does not tell the mental health nurse how to support the service user at a person-centred level. On this basis the nurse needs to pay attention to the service user's narrative and deliver any subsequent interventions through a collaborative and therapeutic relationship (Figure 13.2). These interventions should be:

* underpinned by psychological methods and theory;
* clinically effective and where possible evidenced-based;
* person-centred;
* focused on considering values and meanings.

Further reading

American Psychiatric Association (APA) (2000) *Diagnostic and Statistical Manual of Mental Disorders*, 4th edn, text revision (DSM-IV-TR). Washington, DC: APA.

American Psychiatric Association. DSM-5 Development. Implementation and support for the fifth edition of the Diagnostic and Statistical Manual of Mental Disorders (DSM-5) (http://www.dsm5.org/Pages/Default.aspx).

World Health Organization (WHO) (1992) *The ICD-10 Classification of Mental and Behavioural Disorders: Clinical Descriptions and Diagnostic Guidelines*. Geneva: WHO.

Psychological interventions

Figure 14.1 The practice tree: Psychological interventions

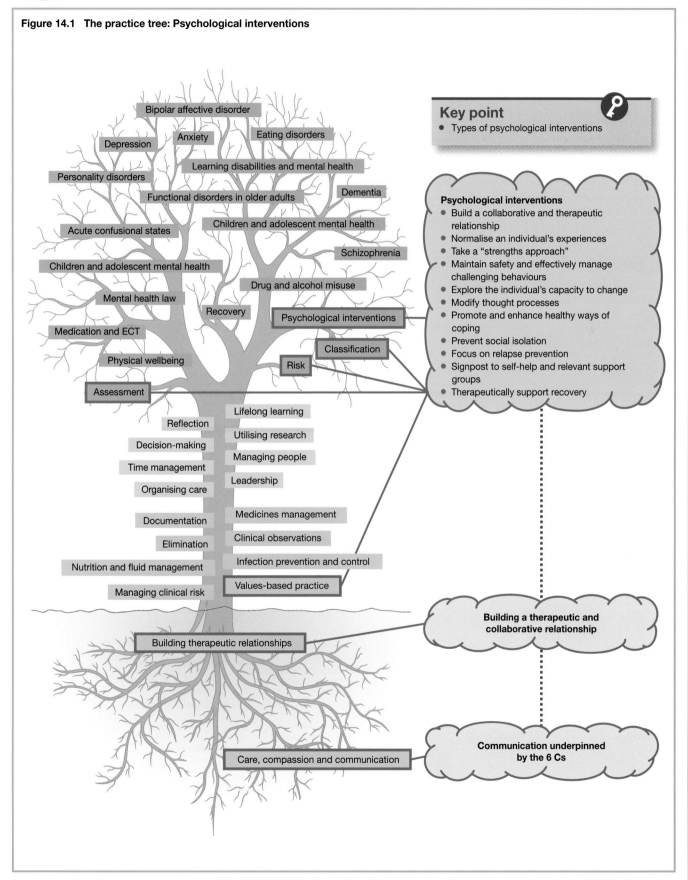

Key point
- Types of psychological interventions

Bipolar affective disorder

Anxiety

Eating disorders

Depression

Learning disabilities and mental health

Personality disorders

Functional disorders in older adults

Dementia

Acute confusional states

Children and adolescent mental health

Schizophrenia

Children and adolescent mental health

Drug and alcohol misuse

Mental health law

Recovery

Psychological interventions

Medication and ECT

Classification

Physical wellbeing

Risk

Assessment

Psychological interventions
- Build a collaborative and therapeutic relationship
- Normalise an individual's experiences
- Take a "strengths approach"
- Maintain safety and effectively manage challenging behaviours
- Explore the individual's capacity to change
- Modify thought processes
- Promote and enhance healthy ways of coping
- Prevent social isolation
- Focus on relapse prevention
- Signpost to self-help and relevant support groups
- Therapeutically support recovery

Lifelong learning

Reflection

Utilising research

Decision-making

Managing people

Time management

Leadership

Organising care

Documentation

Medicines management

Elimination

Clinical observations

Nutrition and fluid management

Infection prevention and control

Managing clinical risk

Values-based practice

Building a therapeutic and collaborative relationship

Building therapeutic relationships

Communication underpinned by the 6 Cs

Care, compassion and communication

Mental Health Nursing at a Glance, First Edition. Grahame Smith. © 2015 John Wiley & Sons, Ltd. Published 2015 by John Wiley & Sons, Ltd.
Companion website: www.ataglanceseries.com/nursing/mentalhealth

Introduction

Mental health nursing practice should be holistic, and taking this into account mental health nurses are professionally required to have the skills, knowledge and values to deliver holistic care that is safe and effective. Psychological interventions are a crucial part of this holistic approach, especially as they aim to improve an individual's biopsychosocial functioning.

Competencies

Mental health nurses are required to:
• Communicate effectively using a wide range of therapeutic strategies and interventions to optimise health and wellbeing.
• Be person-centred and committed to building therapeutic relationships that are enabling and partnership focused.
• Deliver care across settings that is underpinned by a range of evidence-based psychological, psychosocial and other complex therapeutic skills and interventions.
• Deliver care that is systematic, balances the need for safety with positive risk-taking, and promotes recovery.

The context

There is a greater need for mental health nurses to be able to deliver psychological interventions as part of their everyday nursing practice. Certainly clinical guidance related to specific mental disorders will recommend a specific psychological therapy and/or a number of psychological interventions – synonymously known as "psychosocial" interventions. In terms of the wider context of mental health nursing practice psychological interventions are mental health nursing interventions underpinned by psychological methods and theory with the intention of improving biopsychosocial functioning. Delivering the physical health care interventions highlighted in Part 1 would also be underpinned by psychological theories and methods. Whatever the context it is important to recognise that these interventions should be delivered through a therapeutically structured relationship built on the use of good communication skills and a commitment to partnership working.

Psychological therapies

The psychological therapies commonly used in mental health care include the following (see also Figure 14.2):
• cognitive behavioural therapies;
• interpersonal therapy;
• psychodynamic therapy;
• systemic family therapy;
• dialectic behaviour therapy;
• cognitive stimulation;
• motivational enhancement therapy.

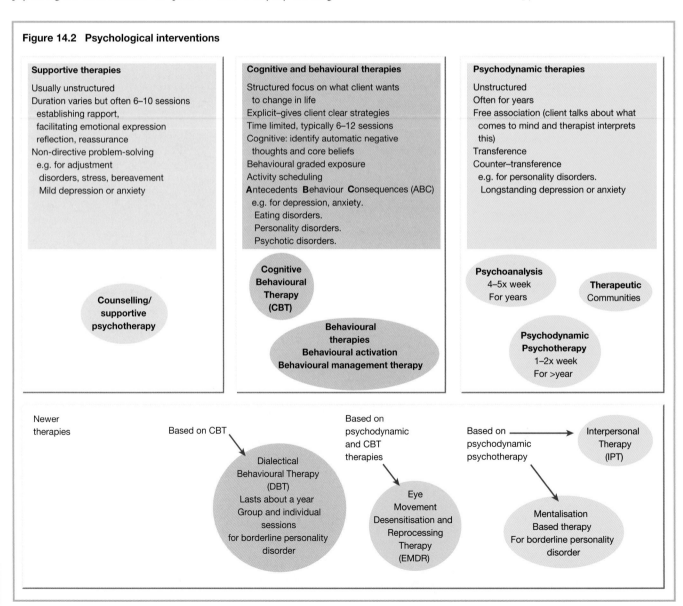

Figure 14.2 Psychological interventions

Supportive therapies

Usually unstructured
Duration varies but often 6–10 sessions
  establishing rapport,
  facilitating emotional expression
  reflection, reassurance
Non-directive problem-solving
  e.g. for adjustment
  disorders, stress, bereavement
  Mild depression or anxiety

Counselling/supportive psychotherapy

Cognitive and behavioural therapies

Structured focus on what client wants
  to change in life
Explicit–gives client clear strategies
Time limited, typically 6–12 sessions
Cognitive: identify automatic negative
  thoughts and core beliefs
Behavioural graded exposure
Activity scheduling
Antecedents **B**ehaviour **C**onsequences (ABC)
  e.g. for depression, anxiety.
  Eating disorders.
  Personality disorders.
  Psychotic disorders.

Cognitive Behavioural Therapy (CBT)

Behavioural therapies
Behavioural activation
Behavioural management therapy

Psychodynamic therapies

Unstructured
Often for years
Free association (client talks about what
  comes to mind and therapist interprets
  this)
Transference
Counter–transference
  e.g. for personality disorders.
  Longstanding depression or anxiety

Psychoanalysis
4–5x week
For years

Therapeutic Communities

Psychodynamic Psychotherapy
1–2x week
For >year

Newer therapies

Based on CBT

Dialectical Behavioural Therapy (DBT)
Lasts about a year
Group and individual sessions
for borderline personality disorder

Based on psychodynamic and CBT therapies

Eye Movement Desensitisation and Reprocessing Therapy (EMDR)

Based on psychodynamic psychotherapy

Interpersonal Therapy (IPT)

Mentalisation Based therapy
For borderline personality disorder

Psychological interventions

Though psychological interventions are usually eclectic and may correspond to more than one psychological therapy or theory they still need to be systematically delivered in way that their effectiveness can be evaluated. Depending on the skill of the mental health nurse (Figure 14.1) they may deliver the following types of psychological interventions:

• Build a collaborative and therapeutic relationship based on a person-centred approach.
• Normalise an individual's experiences of mental distress.
• Take a "strengths approach".
• Maintain safety and effectively manage challenging behaviours.
• Exploring the individual's capacity to change.
• Modifying thought processes – identifying, challenging and replacing negative thoughts.
• Focusing on the individual controlling and regulating their behaviour – promoting and enhancing healthy ways of coping.
• Prevent social isolation and promote social functioning.
• Focus on relapse prevention – early warning signs and self-monitoring of symptoms.
• Signpost to self-help and relevant support groups.
• Therapeutically support recovery.

Being evidence-based

Mental health nurses should deliver psychological interventions that are based on the best evidence available. Taking this into consideration it is also important to recognise that this generalised evidence needs to be situated within the unique nature of the therapeutic relationship. A way of doing this is for the mental health nurse to complement this evidence-based knowledge with knowledge based on knowing the mental health service user they are working with. This type of knowing comes from the use of good communication skills, which focus on truly listening to the mental health service user's story.

Collaboration

Managing risk is an important part of the mental health nurse's role and on this basis being collaborative can be a challenge especially where the mental health nurse has the power to restrict the freedoms of a mental health service user. Unless managed sensitively, this type of power could have an adverse impact upon the therapeutic relationship and any subsequent psychological interventions that are delivered. To address both this power issue and also to continually improve their practice the mental health nurse must actively engage in critical reflection. The process of critically reflecting starts with the mental health nurse using an "open dialogue" approach that focuses on understanding and respecting the service user as a human being rather than as someone to be controlled. The next step is to learn from this approach through structured reflection such as participating in clinical supervision (see Chapter 37).

Further reading

Department of Health (2011) Talking Therapies: A Four-year Plan of Action: A Supporting Document to No Health Without Mental Health: A Cross-government Mental Health Outcomes Strategy for People of All Ages. London: Department of Health.

Gournay, K. (2009) Psychosocial interventions. In: Newell, R. & Gournay, K. (eds), Mental Health Nursing: an Evidence-based Approach, 2nd edn. London: Churchill Livingstone.

Smith, G. (ed.) (2012) Psychological Interventions in Mental Health Nursing. Maidenhead: Open University Press.

Schizophrenia

Figure 15.1 The practice tree: Schizophrenia

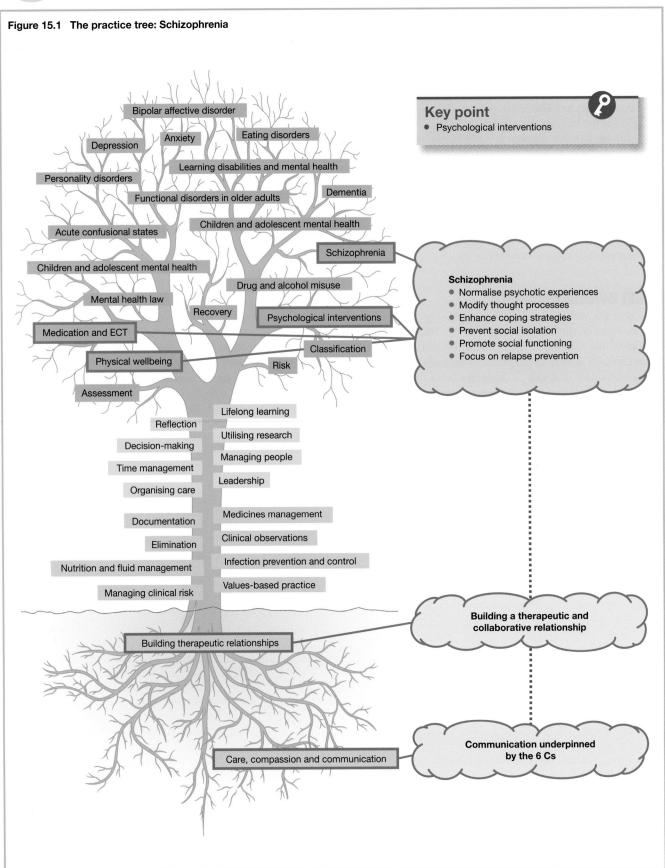

Definitions

Schizophrenia as a medical label originates from the work of Emil Kraepelin (1893) who coined the term "dementia praecox", believing that schizophrenia was an early form of dementia. Paul Eugen Bleuler (1911), building on the work of Kraepelin but moving away from the idea of schizophrenia being an early form of dementia, first used the term schizophrenia – "schiz" meaning "split" and "phren" meaning "mind". Schizophrenia is medically classified as a psychotic disorder; the psychotic disorders also include:

- schizoaffective disorder;
- delusional disorder;
- brief psychotic episodes;
- psychotic depression;
- bipolar affective disorder;
- drug-induced psychosis

Schizophrenia is usually divided into subtypes (although this is changing – see DSM-5):

- disorganised (previously known as hebephrenic);
- catatonic;
- paranoid;
- residual;
- undifferentiated.

A diagnosis of schizophrenia is assigned if at least two of the following symptoms are present for a significant portion of time within a period of 1 month:

- hallucinations;
- delusions;
- disorganised speech;
- catatonic behaviour;
- disorganised behaviour;
- negative symptoms.

Clinical features

In terms of symptoms generally there are positive symptoms, which are distortions of normal functioning:

- hallucinations;
- delusions;
- thought disorders.

And negative symptoms, which are loss of normal functions:

- lack of volition;
- poverty of thought and/or speech.

These symptoms can impact adversely and greatly upon an individual's personal, social and occupational functioning. They can also be experienced over a long period of time with frequent relapses even when antipsychotic medication is being taken.

Risk factors

Around 1% of the population in the UK has a diagnosis of schizophrenia. The causes are not clear, though there are a number of risk factors that may increase the risk of an individual developing the condition:

- presence amongst first-degree relatives;
- age – between the ages of 16 and 40 years;
- gender – early onset for men;
- poor prenatal nutrition;
- obstetric complications;
- low social class;
- substance misuse – stimulants.

Management

Early detection is important in the diagnosis of schizophrenia, and if indicated so is early intervention, especially in the case of a first episode where an individual presents with a very acute and sudden onset. In terms of interventions treatment guidelines recommend:

- cognitive behavioural therapy;
- family interventions;
- art therapy;
- support groups;
- antipsychotic medication.

Psychological interventions

When nursing an individual with a diagnosis of schizophrenia a mental health nurse needs to be able to deliver a range of psychological interventions. Also where there is an increased risk of harm to others and or self, including self-neglect, the nurse should develop appropriate risk management strategies. This does not mean that risky behaviour is an inherent part of the diagnosis of schizophrenia. It may be the case that in the short term the individual may be risky due to experiencing uncontrolled psychotic symptoms where they are struggling to keep themselves safe. In the long term risk is more likely related to an increased risk of mortality due to physical health factors, such as poor diet, little exercise, obesity and smoking. While managing risk the nurse should start to deliver psychological interventions (Figure 15.1), which are shaped by a cognitive behavioural approach:

- Establish a collaborative and therapeutic relationship.
- Normalise psychotic experiences.
- Reduce psychotic symptoms by modifying thought processes and enhancing coping strategies.

Other psychological interventions that have been found to be beneficial include interventions that:

- prevent social isolation;
- promote social functioning;
- focus on relapse prevention;
- alleviate symptoms.

Further reading

Lovejoy, M. (1984) Recovery from schizophrenia: a personal odyssey. *Hospital and Community Psychiatry* **35**: 809–12.

National Institute for Health and Clinical Excellence (NICE) (2009) Schizophrenia: Core Interventions in the Treatment and Management of Schizophrenia in Adults in Primary and Secondary Care (update of NICE clinical guideline 1). London: NICE.

Rusch, N. & Corrigan, P.W. (2002) Motivational interviewing to improve insight and treatment adherence in schizophrenia. *Psychiatric Rehabilitation Journal* **26**(1): 23–32.

16 Depression

Figure 16.1 The practice tree: Depression

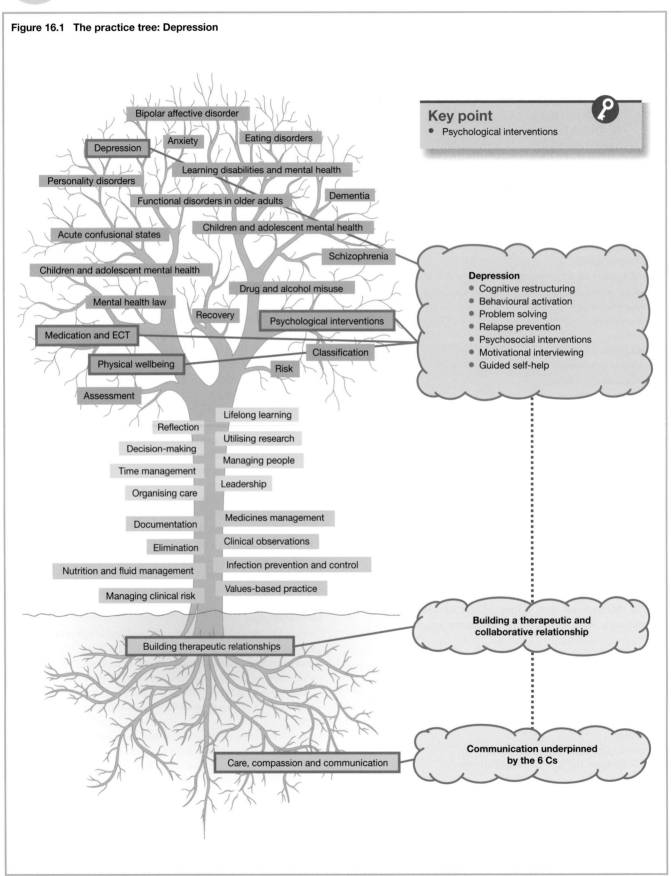

Key point
- Psychological interventions

Depression
- Cognitive restructuring
- Behavioural activation
- Problem solving
- Relapse prevention
- Psychosocial interventions
- Motivational interviewing
- Guided self-help

Bipolar affective disorder

Anxiety

Depression

Eating disorders

Learning disabilities and mental health

Personality disorders

Dementia

Functional disorders in older adults

Children and adolescent mental health

Acute confusional states

Schizophrenia

Children and adolescent mental health

Drug and alcohol misuse

Mental health law

Recovery

Psychological interventions

Medication and ECT

Classification

Physical wellbeing

Risk

Assessment

Lifelong learning

Reflection

Utilising research

Decision-making

Managing people

Time management

Leadership

Organising care

Documentation

Medicines management

Elimination

Clinical observations

Nutrition and fluid management

Infection prevention and control

Managing clinical risk

Values-based practice

Building therapeutic relationships

Building a therapeutic and collaborative relationship

Care, compassion and communication

Communication underpinned by the 6 Cs

Definitions

Depression is classed as a mood disorder where "low mood" is a common symptom. This is not necessarily the same as normal sadness, which may occur following bereavement, a serious physical illness or a traumatic event. The diagnosis of depression is usually described in terms of severity:
- Mild – the symptoms are less intense and they have some impact upon the individual's ability to function.
- Moderate – more of the symptoms are present and they have a greater impact upon the individual's ability to function.
- Severe – the individual has a persistent low mood and the symptoms are distressing to the point that the individual finds it difficult to function.

An individual can have a single or a recurrent depressive episode; a recurrent episode is where an individual has experienced more than one depressive episode. Depression with psychotic symptoms such as hallucinations and delusions is always described as severe. A diagnosis of depression is assigned if at least two of the three core symptoms are present every day for 2 weeks:
- low mood;
- loss of interest;
- low energy.

Associated symptoms include:
- disturbed sleep;
- poor concentration;
- low self-confidence;
- poor appetite;
- suicidal thoughts or acts;
- agitation;
- slowing of movements;
- guilt.

The severity of the episode of depression depends on the:
- number of symptoms;
- the severity of the symptoms and the degree of distress;
- impact upon social functioning.

Clinical features

Individuals can experience a range of cognitive, behavioural and physical symptoms. It is not uncommon for individuals to have negative thoughts about:
- themselves – low self-esteem;
- the world and others;
- their future.

They may also have thoughts that relate to death and suicide.

Risk factors

Depression in all its forms is seen as a common disorder: the estimated lifetime risk can range from 10% to 20%; some estimates can be much higher. This prevalence is also influenced by gender, age and marital status: depression as a diagnosis is higher in females, older adults and individuals living in areas that are classed as deprived. The cause of depression is not clear but there are a number of risk factors that may increase an individual's vulnerability:
- family history of depression;
- psychosocial factors such as loss of employment, parental loss, lack of a confiding relationship;
- severe physical illness;
- childbirth;
- genetic predisposition (theory).

Management

Depression is usually treated within a primary care setting without the need to refer to psychiatric services unless the risk to self and/or others is high, the individual has severe depression that is unresponsive to treatment, or the depressive episode is recurrent or part of a bipolar presentation. In terms of interventions treatment guidelines recommend:
- cognitive behavioural therapy;
- interpersonal therapy;
- guided self-help;
- self-help groups;
- structured physical activity;
- behavioural activation;
- antidepressants;
- ECT in severe cases.

Psychological interventions

Mental health nurses work in a variety of settings and on this basis they can work with individuals who have been diagnosed with mild, moderate or severe depression. Therefore it is important that mental health nurses follow a stepped care model that is designed to indicate the choice of intervention by the severity of the depressive episode. Before the nurse delivers any specific psychological interventions they will need to ensure that they have built an effective therapeutic relationship; they will also need to manage any identified risk and/or any comorbid conditions. Depending on the skill of the nurse the types of interventions (Figure 16.1) they may deliver are:
- cognitive restructuring;
- behavioural activation;
- problem solving;
- relapse prevention;
- psychosocial interventions;
- motivational interviewing;
- guided self-help.

Further reading

Bortolotti, B., Menchetti, M., Bellini, F., Montaguti, M.B. & Berardi, D. (2008) Psychological interventions for major depression in primary care: a meta-analytic review of randomized controlled trials. *General Hospital Psychiatry* **30**(4): 293–302.

Lovell, K. & Richards, D. (2008) *A Recovery Programme for Depression*. London: Rethink.

National Institute of Clinical Excellence (NICE) (2009) *The Treatment and Management of Depression in Adults*, updated edn. London: British Psychological Society and Royal College of Psychiatrists.

17 Bipolar affective disorder

Figure 17.1 The practice tree: Bipolar affective disorder

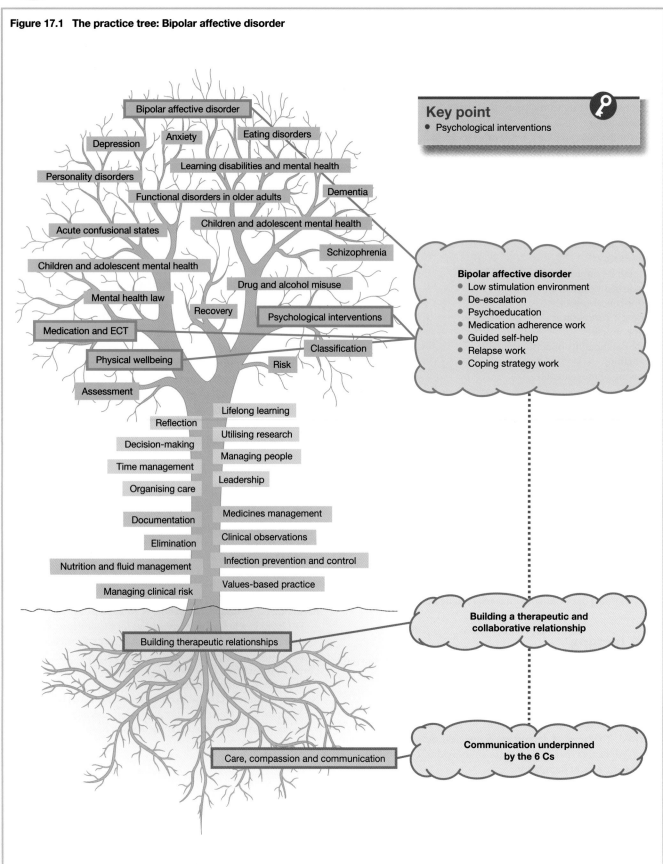

Definitions

Bipolar affective disorder, which is also historically known as manic depression, is classified as a psychosis. Bipolar disorder, unlike a unipolar disorder such as major depression, is a disorder where an individual's mood state fluctuates between low and high mood states. This is not just a case of someone feeling sad and then happy; these mood states can significantly impact on an individual's ability to function at an everyday level. Bipolar disorder is classified in terms of episodes:

- depressive episode – (see Chapter 16);
- manic episode – an individual may feel full of energy and have grandiose ideas about themselves;
- hypomanic – less severe than a manic episode;
- mixed – where manic and depressive features present at the same time or alternate rapidly.

and types:

- bipolar I – one or more manic episodes;
- bipolar II – recurrent severe depression and hypomanic episodes;
- rapid cycling – more than four mood swings in a 12-month period;
- cyclothymia – enduring mood fluctuations that are not as severe as in full bipolar disorder.

In terms of manic episodes then bipolar I disorder is viewed as being more severe. A diagnosis of bipolar I disorder is usually assigned if the individual:

- has had at least one manic or mixed episode for at least one week in duration
- their symptoms cause significant distress or impairment.

Clinical features

The key feature of bipolar affective disorder is usually the fluctuation in mood states, especially the presence of elevated or a high mood state, mania and to a lesser degree hypomania. During this elevated mood state an individual may feel irritable and:

- have an inflated sense of self-esteem and grandiose ideas;
- have a decreased need for sleep;
- talk rapidly with racing thoughts;
- be easily distracted and over-active;
- have delusions and hallucinations – in mania only;
- they may also increasingly engage in risky behaviours such as sexual overactivity, dangerous driving and reckless spending.

Risk factors

It is estimated in terms of lifetime prevalence that around 4% of individuals will experience a bipolar affective disorder, more likely cyclothymia. Though the causes are not clear there is an increasing view that there is a strong genetic element to the disorder. Risk factors that may increase the risk of an individual developing the condition include:

- presence amongst first-degree relatives;
- higher social class;
- life events such as childhood abuse and loss;
- sleep problems;
- age – early twenties;
- gender – bipolar II more prevalent in women;
- severe physical illness – stroke.

Management

The first line of treatment for bipolar affective disorder focuses on psychiatric medication that reduces the severity of the symptoms, stabilises mood fluctuations and prevents relapse. Treatment guidelines also recommend:

- cognitive behavioural therapy;
- family-focused therapy;
- psychoeducation;
- interpersonal therapy;
- ECT in severe mania or depression.

Psychological interventions

Individuals diagnosed with a bipolar affective disorder may require rapid access to support especially when they are experiencing severe symptoms. At this juncture managing risk to self and/or others may be a priority particularly when an individual's mood is elevated. In this case it is important to provide an environment that is low in stimulation, ensure that the individual's dietary and fluid needs are met, and only use physical restraint as a last option – de-escalation techniques are always preferable. The mental health nurse (Figure 17.1) would also need to:

- build a collaborative and therapeutic relationship;
- provide psychoeducation including medication adherence work;
- signpost to self-help and relevant support groups;
- relapse work – early warning signs and self-monitoring of symptoms;
- coping strategy work.

It is also important to recognise that any psychological intervention would need to be tailored for the individual, especially if they are also experiencing severe depressive episodes (see Chapter 16). Due to the type of medications that are prescribed to treat bipolar affective disorder individuals who are being treated should also have an annual physical health review.

Further reading

Crowe, M., Whitehead, L., Wilson, L., Carlyle, D., O'Brien, A., Inder, M. & Joyce, P. (2010) Disorder-specific psychosocial interventions for bipolar disorder: A systematic review of the evidence for mental health nursing practice. *International Journal of Nursing Studies* **47**: 896–908.

Dahlqvist Jönsson, P., Skärsäter, I., Wijk, H. & Danielson, E. (2011) Experience of living with a family member with bipolar disorder. *International Journal of Mental Health Nursing* **20**: 29–37.

National Institute for Health and Clinical Excellence (NICE) (2006) Bipolar Disorder: The Management of Bipolar Disorder in Adults, Children and Adolescents, in Primary and Secondary Care – Clinical Guideline 38. London: NICE.

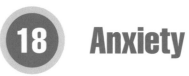 **Anxiety**

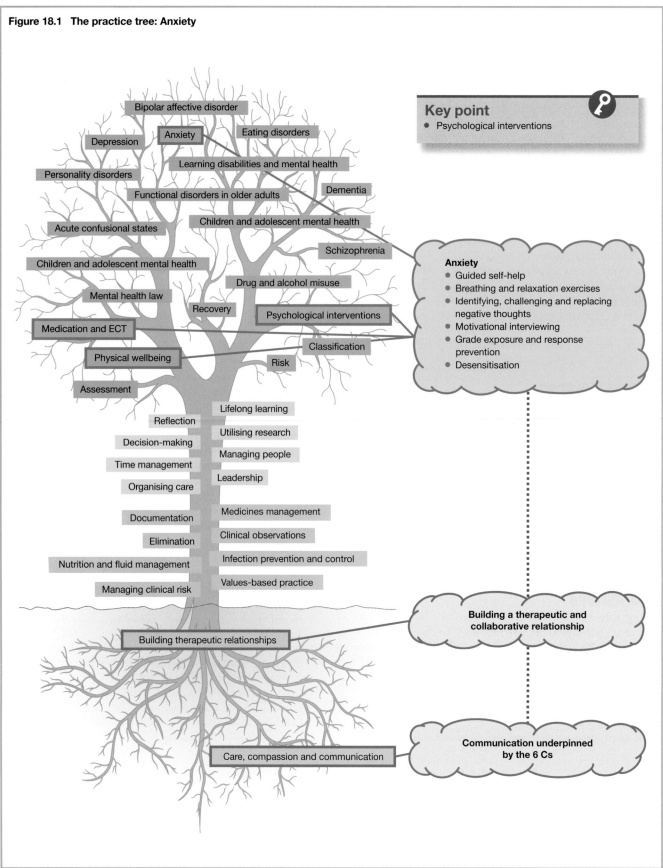

Figure 18.1 The practice tree: Anxiety

Bipolar affective disorder

Anxiety

Depression

Eating disorders

Personality disorders

Learning disabilities and mental health

Functional disorders in older adults

Dementia

Acute confusional states

Children and adolescent mental health

Children and adolescent mental health

Schizophrenia

Drug and alcohol misuse

Mental health law

Recovery

Psychological interventions

Medication and ECT

Classification

Physical wellbeing

Risk

Assessment

Lifelong learning

Reflection

Utilising research

Decision-making

Managing people

Time management

Leadership

Organising care

Documentation

Medicines management

Elimination

Clinical observations

Nutrition and fluid management

Infection prevention and control

Managing clinical risk

Values-based practice

Building therapeutic relationships

Care, compassion and communication

Key point
- Psychological interventions

Anxiety
- Guided self-help
- Breathing and relaxation exercises
- Identifying, challenging and replacing negative thoughts
- Motivational interviewing
- Grade exposure and response prevention
- Desensitisation

Building a therapeutic and collaborative relationship

Communication underpinned by the 6 Cs

Mental Health Nursing at a Glance, First Edition. Grahame Smith. © 2015 John Wiley & Sons, Ltd. Published 2015 by John Wiley & Sons, Ltd.
Companion website: www.ataglanceseries.com/nursing/mentalhealth

Definitions

When we are anxious we may feel frightened, or apprehensive; we may also feel physically tense with a sense that our heart is beating faster than normal. It is not unusual to feel anxious and in some cases it can be quite useful especially when your body needs to be prepared to "fight or run". Where anxiety becomes problematic is when it interferes with our ability to function. This may happen when there are persistent and enduring feelings of dread, apprehension or uneasiness even when there is no recognisable danger. Anxiety disorders can be divided into three main types:

- Generalised Anxiety Disorder (GAD) – a generalised and persistent anxiety lasting at least longer than 3 weeks.
- Panic Disorder – recurrent and severe panic attacks that occur unpredictably (a minimum of three panic attacks over a 3-week period).
- Phobia – a fear that can become panic in specific situations, such as certain places, objects, animals, at heights, and in closed or open spaces.

 Other related disorders include:

- Obsessive Compulsive Disorder (OCD) – recurrent obsessional thoughts or compulsive acts with a frequency greater than 1 hour per day and with duration of at least 2 weeks.
- Post-Traumatic Stress Disorder (PTSD) – a fearful response to threatening and/or catastrophic events, which is re-experienced through upsetting thoughts or memories and leads to avoiding certain situations. The individual may have difficulty sleeping, feel irritable and may also have difficulty concentrating (the symptoms must have lasted for more than 1 month).

Clinical features

Individuals with an anxiety disorder can experience a range of cognitive, behavioural and physical symptoms depending on the condition:

- fear and worry;
- increased vigilance;
- irritability and restlessness;
- poor concentration;
- sleeping difficulties;
- physical tension;
- hyperactivity;
- palpitations;
- abdominal discomfit and nausea;
- hot flushes;
- outbursts of anger;
- ruminating thoughts and compulsions.

Risk factors

The prevalence of anxiety disorders in the general population is around 6% at any one time, with GAD being the most common anxiety disorder. The causes of anxiety disorders are not clear but there are a number of risk factors that may increase an individual's vulnerability:

- gender – more common in women;
- age – more common in younger and middle-aged adults;
- drug misuse – can heighten anxiety states;
- family history;
- life events such as childhood abuse, loss of employment, parental loss, excessive demands or high expectations;
- severe physical illness.

Management

Anxiety disorders, similarly to the treatment of depression, are usually treated within a primary care setting. Again, like in the treatment for depression, a stepped care model is followed. In terms of specific interventions these are dependent on the condition and the individual's preference. Treatment guidelines recommend:

- cognitive behavioural therapy;
- behavioural therapy;
- medication such as selective serotonin reuptake inhibitors;
- interpersonal therapy;
- group therapy;
- psychodynamic therapy;
- mindfulness approaches
- systemic therapy;
- eye movement desensitisation;
- relaxation techniques.

Psychological Interventions

Mental health nurses work in a variety of settings and they will encounter individuals who have been diagnosed with an anxiety disorder, both as a disorder on its own or as a comorbid disorder. It is not uncommon for an anxiety disorder to be comorbid with other disorders such as depression, substance misuse or another anxiety disorder. Similar to the treatment for depression it is important that mental health nurses follow a stepped care model that is designed to indicate the choice of intervention. Risk needs to be managed as part of the delivery of any psychological intervention as well as ensuring that an effective therapeutic relationship has been built. Depending on the skill and training of the nurse the types of interventions (Figure 18.1) the nurse may deliver are:

- guided self-help;
- breathing and relaxation exercises;
- identifying, challenging and replacing negative thoughts;
- motivational interviewing;
- grade exposure and response prevention;
- desensitisation.

Further reading

Hunot, V., Churchill, R., Teixeira, V. & Silva de Lima, M. (2007) Psychological therapies for generalised anxiety disorder. *Cochrane Database of Systematic Reviews* issue 1; CD001848.

National Institute of Clinical Excellence (NICE) (2005) *Obsessive-Compulsive Disorder: Core Interventions in the Treatment of Obsessive-Compulsive Disorder and Body Dysmorphic Disorder.* London: British Psychological Society and Royal College of Psychiatrists.

National Institute of Clinical Excellence (NICE) (2011) *Generalised Anxiety Disorder and Panic Disorder (with or without Agoraphobia) in Adults: Management in Primary, Secondary and Community Care*, partial update. London: British Psychological Society and Royal College of Psychiatrists.

19 Eating disorders

Figure 19.1 The practice tree: Eating disorders

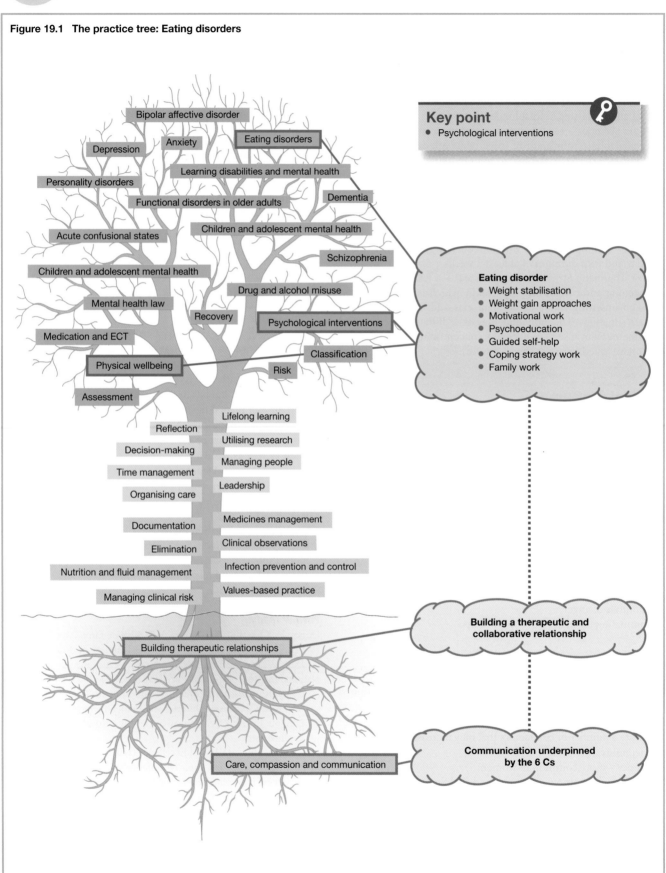

Key point
- Psychological interventions

Eating disorder
- Weight stabilisation
- Weight gain approaches
- Motivational work
- Psychoeducation
- Guided self-help
- Coping strategy work
- Family work

Bipolar affective disorder
Eating disorders
Anxiety
Depression
Learning disabilities and mental health
Personality disorders
Dementia
Functional disorders in older adults
Children and adolescent mental health
Acute confusional states
Schizophrenia
Children and adolescent mental health
Drug and alcohol misuse
Mental health law
Recovery
Psychological interventions
Medication and ECT
Classification
Physical wellbeing
Risk
Assessment

Lifelong learning
Reflection
Utilising research
Decision-making
Managing people
Time management
Leadership
Organising care
Documentation
Medicines management
Elimination
Clinical observations
Nutrition and fluid management
Infection prevention and control
Managing clinical risk
Values-based practice

Building therapeutic relationships

Building a therapeutic and collaborative relationship

Care, compassion and communication

Communication underpinned by the 6 Cs

Mental Health Nursing at a Glance, First Edition. Grahame Smith. © 2015 John Wiley & Sons, Ltd. Published 2015 by John Wiley & Sons, Ltd.
Companion website: www.ataglanceseries.com/nursing/mentalhealth

Definitions

The term "eating disorder" indicates that an individual has abnormal eating habits. This may include not eating enough food and eating food in excess. These eating habits also impact adversely on the individual's health and wellbeing. The most common eating disorders are:

- anorexia nervosa – morbid fear of fatness;
- bulimia nervosa – morbid fear of fatness with binge eating;
- binge eating disorder – binge eating without purging.

An eating disorder diagnosis is usually assigned if the individual in the case of:

- anorexia nervosa – has a morbid fear of fatness with a distorted body image, is deliberately losing weight (a specifically low body mass index, BMI), and has amenorrhoea;
- bulimia nervosa – has a morbid fear of fatness and a preoccupation with body weight, is binge eating on large amounts of food and is trying to prevent weight gain through such behaviours as vomiting and misusing laxatives;
- binge eating disorder – is binge eating without purging and this behaviour is leading to obesity (measured by BMI).

Clinical features

The eating disorders, especially anorexia nervosa and bulimia nervosa, are characterised by a preoccupation with weight and body image. Purging and binge eating can also be present in anorexia nervosa. Other features include:

- self-conscious about eating in public;
- dieting;
- excessive exercise;
- constipation;
- emaciation;
- dry skin;
- bradycardia and hypotension.

The clinical features of bulimia nervosa also include:

- craving for food;
- fluctuating weight;
- fasting;
- excessive exercise;
- intense self-loathing especially after bingeing;
- amenorrhoea;
- acute oesophageal tears – vomiting related.

Risk factors

Eating disorders primarily affect females, with anorexia and bulimia nervosa being three times more common in females than males. The prevalence rates for eating disorders range from 10% to 20% of the population, with 1–3% having a specific diagnosis. The causes of eating disorders are not clear though there are risk factors that may increase the risk of an individual developing the condition such as:

- Presence amongst first-degree relatives or a first-degree relative who has an anxiety disorder, depression, or an obsessional personality, or in the case of bulimia nervosa has a substance misuse diagnosis.

- Age – early adolescence in anorexia nervosa; late teens in bulimia nervosa.
- Low self-esteem.
- Difficulty in expressing emotions – anorexia nervosa.
- Impulsive – bulimia nervosa.
- An upbringing where weight and food are over-valued.
- Bullied about their weight.
- Life events – childhood abuse and loss.

Management

The first-line treatment for adolescents with anorexia nervosa is family therapy, and for adults there are a number of therapies that can be offered, which include:

- cognitive behavioural therapy;
- interpersonal therapy;
- psychodynamic therapy;
- family therapy;
- medication – where depression is comorbid.

The first line of treatment for bulimia nervosa is usually cognitive behavioural therapy or interpersonal therapy; antidepressants can also be prescribed where depression is comorbid. In binge eating disorder treatment usually consists of cognitive behavioural therapy, exercise and nutritional education.

Psychological interventions

Individuals diagnosed with an eating disorder are usually treated outside the in-patient setting. In the case of anorexia nervosa treatment within an in-patient setting may be required where there is a significant risk to self; this can be due to suicidal thoughts or the physical impact of the disorder. The mental health nurse (Figure 19.1) may need to stabilise the individual's physical condition before instigating the following psychological interventions:

- build a collaborative and therapeutic relationship;
- motivational work;
- psychoeducation and guided self-help;
- behavioural work – weight gain;
- coping strategy work;
- family work.

Further reading

Fox, A.P., Larkin, M. & Leung, N. (2011) The personal meaning of eating disorder symptoms: an interpretative phenomenological analysis. *Journal of Health Psychology* **16**: 116–25.

National Institute for Clinical Excellence (NICE) (2004) Eating Disorders: Core Interventions in the Treatment and Management of Anorexia Nervosa, Bulimia Nervosa and Related Eating Disorders – Clinical Guideline 9. London: NICE.

Wright, K.M. (2010) Therapeutic relationship: Developing a new understanding for nurses and care workers within an eating disorder unit. *International Journal of Mental Health Nursing* **19**: 154–61.

Personality disorders

Figure 20.1 The practice tree: Personality disorders

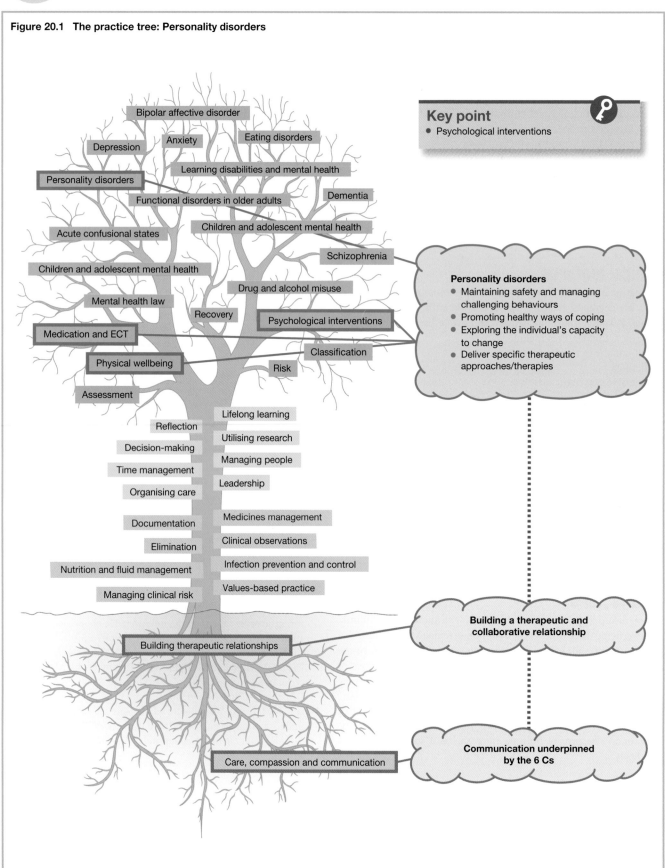

Bipolar affective disorder

Anxiety

Eating disorders

Depression

Learning disabilities and mental health

Personality disorders

Functional disorders in older adults

Dementia

Children and adolescent mental health

Acute confusional states

Schizophrenia

Children and adolescent mental health

Drug and alcohol misuse

Mental health law

Recovery

Psychological interventions

Medication and ECT

Classification

Physical wellbeing

Risk

Assessment

Lifelong learning

Reflection

Utilising research

Decision-making

Managing people

Time management

Leadership

Organising care

Documentation

Medicines management

Elimination

Clinical observations

Nutrition and fluid management

Infection prevention and control

Managing clinical risk

Values-based practice

Building therapeutic relationships

Care, compassion and communication

Key point
- Psychological interventions

Personality disorders
- Maintaining safety and managing challenging behaviours
- Promoting healthy ways of coping
- Exploring the individual's capacity to change
- Deliver specific therapeutic approaches/therapies

Building a therapeutic and collaborative relationship

Communication underpinned by the 6 Cs

Mental Health Nursing at a Glance, First Edition. Grahame Smith. © 2015 John Wiley & Sons, Ltd. Published 2015 by John Wiley & Sons, Ltd.
Companion website: www.ataglanceseries.com/nursing/mentalhealth

Definitions

It can be argued that personality is unique to the individual and that it cannot be measured or quantified. Others would argue that there are specific traits that can be measured and generalised in a way that we can talk about personality types. By having a measured sense of normal personality this can lead to having a sense of what is not the accepted norm, and when this process is medicalised this in turn can lead to a personality disorder diagnosis being applied. Personality disorders can be described as behaviour patterns that are enduring and deeply ingrained, that distinctly deviate from what would be culturally expected, and that lead to distress to self and/or others. Personality disorders are categorised in terms of three main clusters or nine types; the methods of categorising personality disorders are similar though some names are slightly different, and narcissistic personality disorder is not included when using types. The three main clusters and types are:

- Cluster A – paranoid, schizoid and schizotypal.
- Cluster B – antisocial (type: dissocial), borderline (type: emotionally unstable), histrionic and narcissistic (not included in types).
- Cluster C – avoidant (type: anxious), dependent, obsessive compulsive (type: anankastic).

A personality disorder is diagnosed not just in terms of whether specific traits are present but also in terms of how severe those traits are, whether or not there is significant risk to self and/or others, and how they impact upon the individual's social functioning.

Clinical features

It is not uncommon for an individual to exhibit traits that can fall into more than one personality disorder cluster and/or type. It is also not uncommon for a personality disorder to be either comorbid with another mental health disorder or to be misdiagnosed. On this basis it is important that a full and comprehensive assessment is undertaken and that any comorbid disorders are also identified and treated. The following is a list of some of the personality traits that an individual diagnosed with a specific personality disorder can exhibit:

- paranoid – suspicious and excessively sensitive;
- schizoid – emotional coldness, little interest in other people;
- schizotypal – odd beliefs and unusual appearance;
- borderline – instability of mood, impulsive;
- histrionic – excessive attention seeking;
- narcissistic – grandiose and arrogant;
- antisocial – disregard of self and others;
- avoidant – feelings of inadequacy;
- dependent – submissive behaviour;
- obsessive-compulsive – a preoccupation with orderliness.

Risk factors

The prevalence rate for personality disorders can range from 2% to 13%; some studies use an average of 5% for the general population. The rate is significantly higher in populations of individuals being treated for a mental health disorder. The causes of personality disorders are not clear though there are risk factors that may increase the risk of an individual developing the condition, such as:

- problems in early childhood – abuse, neglect and trauma;
- family history, including similar personality traits within the family;
- presence of other mental health problems;
- lack of adequate support for childhood traumas;
- unhealthy coping strategies.

Management

The management of individuals with a personality disorder has in the past been influenced by concerns over treatability. There are now a number of treatments that show promise for individuals diagnosed with a personality disorder especially where they are diagnosed with either a borderline or an antisocial personality disorder. These include:

- cognitive behaviour therapy – group and individual;
- behavioural approaches;
- mentalisation-based approaches;
- dialectic behaviour therapy;
- therapeutic community treatments.

Psychological interventions

Mental health nurses working with individuals diagnosed with a personality disorder need to consider risk especially in terms of suicide. Where the individual is a risk to self and/or others the mental health nurse first implements psychological interventions that manage this identified risk; these could include the use of medication. At the same time the mental health nurse works with the individual in the process of building a therapeutic relationship. In the long term this relationship will be a vehicle for the utilisation of specific therapeutic approaches that can assist the individual in regulating their own behaviour. Depending on the skill of the nurse the types of psychological interventions (Figure 20.1) the nurse may deliver include:

- Interventions that maintain safety and effectively manage challenging behaviours – boundary setting.
- Focusing on the individual controlling and regulating their behaviour – promoting healthy ways of coping.
- Exploring the individual's capacity to change – motivational interviewing and pre-therapy work.
- Delivering specific therapeutic approaches/therapies.

Further reading

James, P.D. & Cowman, S. (2007) Psychiatric nurses' knowledge, experience and attitudes towards clients with borderline personality disorder. *Journal of Psychiatric and Mental Health Nursing* **14**(7): 670–8.

Livesley, W.J. (2005) Principles and strategies for treating personality disorder. *Canadian Journal of Psychiatry* **50**(8): 442–50.

National Institute for Mental Health in England (2003) *Personality Disorder: No Longer a Diagnosis of Exclusion. Policy Implementation Guidance for the Development of Services for People with Personality Disorder.* London: NIMHE.

Learning disabilities and mental health

Figure 21.1 The practice tree: Learning disabilities and mental health

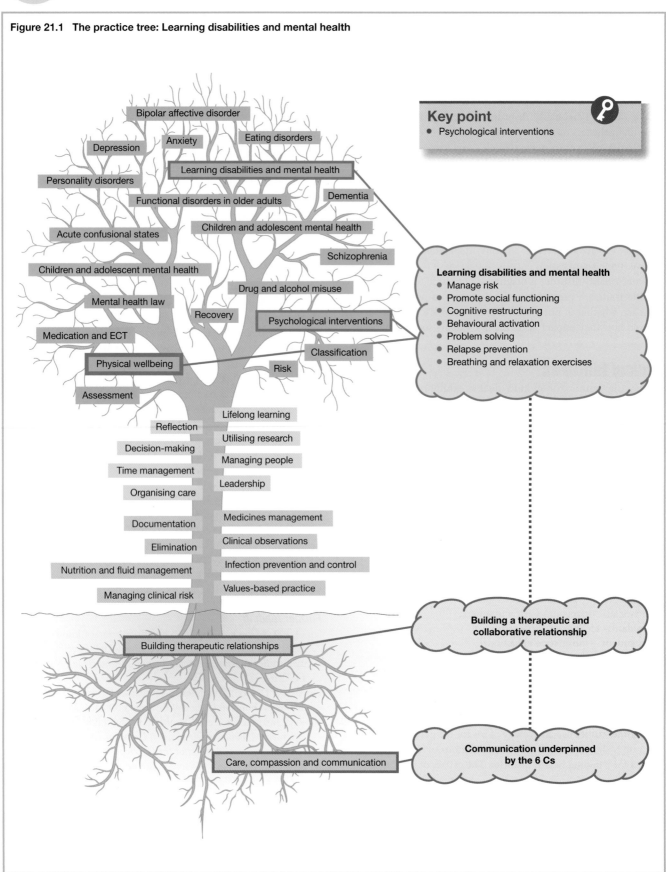

Key point
- Psychological interventions

Learning disabilities and mental health
- Manage risk
- Promote social functioning
- Cognitive restructuring
- Behavioural activation
- Problem solving
- Relapse prevention
- Breathing and relaxation exercises

Bipolar affective disorder
Anxiety
Eating disorders
Depression
Personality disorders
Learning disabilities and mental health
Functional disorders in older adults
Dementia
Acute confusional states
Children and adolescent mental health
Schizophrenia
Children and adolescent mental health
Drug and alcohol misuse
Mental health law
Recovery
Psychological interventions
Medication and ECT
Classification
Physical wellbeing
Risk
Assessment
Lifelong learning
Reflection
Utilising research
Decision-making
Managing people
Time management
Leadership
Organising care
Documentation
Medicines management
Elimination
Clinical observations
Nutrition and fluid management
Infection prevention and control
Managing clinical risk
Values-based practice

Building therapeutic relationships

Building a therapeutic and collaborative relationship

Care, compassion and communication

Communication underpinned by the 6 Cs

Mental Health Nursing at a Glance, First Edition. Grahame Smith. © 2015 John Wiley & Sons, Ltd. Published 2015 by John Wiley & Sons, Ltd.
Companion website: www.ataglanceseries.com/nursing/mentalhealth

Definitions

Learning disabilities, sometimes known as intellectual disabilities and formerly classified as mental retardation (DSM-IV), can be described as a reduced intellectual ability that has onset before adulthood and can adversely affect an individual's social functioning. A learning disability is classed as:

- profound – IQ below 20;
- severe – IQ between 20 and 34;
- moderate – IQ between 35 and 49;
- mild – IQ between 50 and 69.

The majority of individuals with a learning disability do not have a comorbid mental health disorder, though there is an increased likelihood of being diagnosed with the following disorders:

- depression;
- obsessive-compulsive disorder;
- phobia;
- schizophrenia;
- mania.

Diagnosing a specific mental health disorder may be difficult in the case of an individual who has profound communication difficulties or where symptoms that would usually be viewed as being related to an underlying mental health disorder are instead viewed as learning disability behaviours.

Clinical features

Individuals with a learning disability and a comorbid mental health disorder are usually described as having a dual diagnosis. The problem with the use of this term is that it is vague; but also the term dual diagnosis can refer to any individual who has more than one diagnosis whether it be a mental health, learning disability or physical condition. Individuals can experience a range of cognitive, behavioural and physical symptoms, which include:

- self-harm;
- aggression;
- inappropriate sexual behaviour;
- disturbed sleep;
- restlessness;
- compulsions;
- tearfulness;
- hallucinations;
- paranoid delusions.

Risk factors

The prevalence of individuals with a learning disability is about 1.5% of the general population. Among the population of individuals with a learning disability there is increased prevalence of mental health problems, which can range from 20 to 40% at any one time. The causes of these mental health problems are not clear but there are a number of risk factors that may increase an individual's vulnerability:

- unemployment;
- discrimination;
- abuse;
- poverty;
- drug and alcohol problems;
- sensory impairments.

Management

Treating individuals with a learning disability and a mental health disorder is similar to the treatment delivered for a individual without a learning disability. Depending on the presenting issues, specific treatments could include:

- behavioural approaches;
- cognitive behavioural therapy;
- antidepressants;
- interpersonal therapy;
- psychodynamic therapy;
- relaxation techniques;
- psychoeducation;
- art therapy;
- antipsychotic medication.

Psychological interventions

Individuals with a learning disability may have an existing package of support in place prior to being diagnosed with a comorbid mental health disorder. Where this is the case the mental health nurse needs to tailor any subsequent psychological interventions in a way that complements this existing care package. This may mean that the mental health nurse has to work across agencies and different settings, both as someone who is directly delivering care and as someone who is supporting and advising others who are delivering care. Depending on the skill of the nurse the types of psychological interventions (Figure 21.1) the nurse may deliver include:

- build a collaborative and therapeutic relationship;
- manage risk;
- promote social functioning;
- cognitive restructuring;
- behavioural activation;
- problem solving;
- relapse prevention;
- breathing and relaxation exercises.

Further reading

Department of Health (2009) *Valuing People Now: A New Three Year Strategy for People with Learning Disabilities*. London: Department of Health.

Raghavan, R., Marshall, M., Lockwood, A. & Duggan, L. (2004) Assessing the needs of people with learning disabilities and mental illness: development of the learning disability version of the Cardinal Needs Schedule (LDCNS). *Journal of Intellectual Disability Research* **48**(1): 25–36.

Raghavan, R. & Patel, P. (2005) *Learning Disabilities and Mental Health: A Nursing Perspective*. Oxford: Blackwell.

22 Functional disorders in older adults

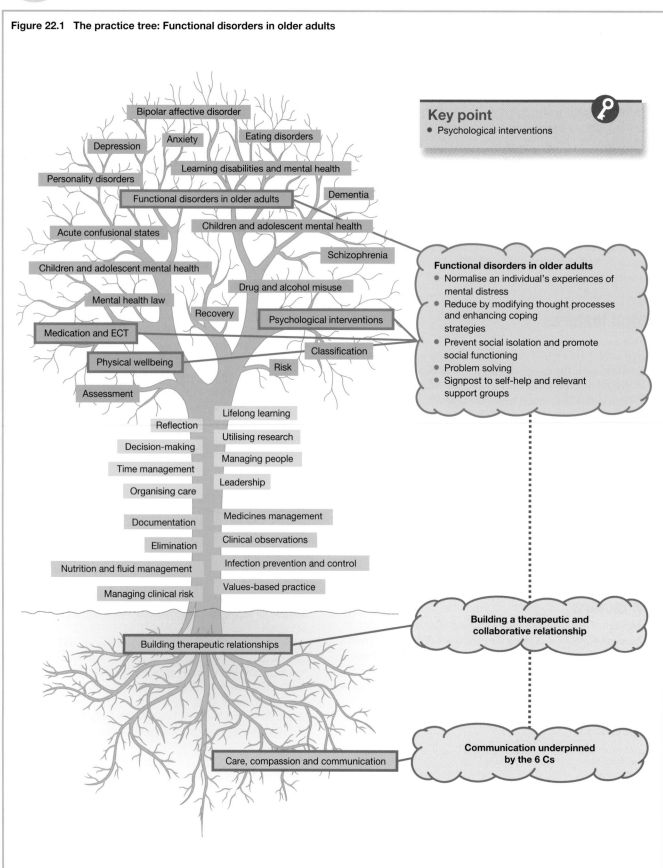

Figure 22.1 The practice tree: Functional disorders in older adults

Bipolar affective disorder

Anxiety

Eating disorders

Depression

Learning disabilities and mental health

Personality disorders

Functional disorders in older adults

Dementia

Acute confusional states

Children and adolescent mental health

Children and adolescent mental health

Schizophrenia

Drug and alcohol misuse

Mental health law

Recovery

Psychological interventions

Medication and ECT

Classification

Physical wellbeing

Risk

Assessment

Lifelong learning

Reflection

Utilising research

Decision-making

Managing people

Time management

Leadership

Organising care

Documentation

Medicines management

Elimination

Clinical observations

Nutrition and fluid management

Infection prevention and control

Managing clinical risk

Values-based practice

Building therapeutic relationships

Care, compassion and communication

Key point
- Psychological interventions

Functional disorders in older adults
- Normalise an individual's experiences of mental distress
- Reduce by modifying thought processes and enhancing coping strategies
- Prevent social isolation and promote social functioning
- Problem solving
- Signpost to self-help and relevant support groups

Building a therapeutic and collaborative relationship

Communication underpinned by the 6 Cs

Mental Health Nursing at a Glance, First Edition. Grahame Smith. © 2015 John Wiley & Sons, Ltd. Published 2015 by John Wiley & Sons, Ltd.
Companion website: www.ataglanceseries.com/nursing/mentalhealth

Definitions

As individuals live longer we have an increasingly aging population, and mental health nurses need to be able to respond effectively to this change. Historically mental health services have been demarcated as services for individuals under the age of 65 and services for individuals over the age of 65. This artificial division is now changing with a focus on providing services that are needs-led. In terms of functional disorders older adults have similar needs to younger adults and on this basis they should be given a similar level of care.

Generally a functional disorder is different from an organic disorder in that organic disorders result from an identified biological cause whereas in functional disorders there is no apparent biological cause. Functional disorders in older adults include:

- personality disorders;
- depression;
- anxiety disorders;
- mania;
- psychotic disorders.

The assessment, diagnosis and management of these functional disorders is the same for older adults as for younger adults.

Clinical features

The normal aging process may mean that an individual experiences a number of changes, which can be physical, psychological, social and spiritual. These changes and also how society generally views the aging process can have an impact upon the presentation, diagnosis and treatment of a given functional disorder:

- Older adults are less likely to report low mood or suicidal thoughts.
- Depression tends to be viewed as part of the aging process and due to this the appropriate treatment is not always given.
- Certain psychiatric medications are to be used with caution where there is a coexisting physical illness.
- Traumatic events such as a fall or a physical illness such as a stroke can lead to the onset of a functional disorder.
- Mania is more likely to present in terms of irritability rather than overt elation.
- Older adults are at a higher risk of completed suicide than younger adults.

Risk factors

Depression and anxiety disorders are the most common functional disorders diagnosed in older adults; the prevalence rates with all the functional disorders, except bipolar disorder, increase with age. Similar to functional disorders in younger adults the cause of functional disorders in older adults is not clear but there are a number of risk factors that may increase an individual's vulnerability:

- the presence of a dementia increases the risk of depression;
- physical illness increases the risk of depression or mania;
- being socially isolated increases the risk of depression or a psychotic disorder;
- being in a nursing home or residential care increases the risk of depression;
- being a carer for someone with dementia increases the risk of depression;
- traumatic events increase the risk of an anxiety disorder;
- loss can increase the risk of depression or a psychotic disorder.

Management

Treatment is dependent on the functional disorder and its presentation, the individual's circumstances and their specific needs. Ensuring the individual is not socially isolated is a key part of the recovery process. In terms of interventions treatment guidelines recommend:

- cognitive behavioural therapy – individual or group;
- treat any underlying physical illnesses;
- guided self-help;
- psychoeducation;
- group therapy;
- structured physical activity;
- behavioural activation;
- relaxation techniques;
- psychiatric medication;
- ECT in severe cases (depression).

Psychological interventions

When nursing older adults diagnosed with a functional disorder it is important that the individual is thoroughly assessed; this includes establishing whether there is an underlying physical condition. Also the risk assessment and management process needs to be sensitive to the increased risk of completed suicide in older adults. Depending on the skill of the nurse the types of interventions (Figure 22.1) they may deliver are:

- establish a collaborative therapeutic relationship;
- normalise an individual's experiences of mental distress;
- reduce by modifying thought processes and enhancing coping strategies;
- prevent social isolation and promote social functioning;
- problem solving;
- signpost to self-help and relevant support groups.

Further reading

Goldberg, S.E., Whittamore, K.H., Harwood, R.H., Bradshaw, L.E., Gladman, J.R.F. & Jones, R.G. (2012) The prevalence of mental health problems among older adults admitted as an emergency to a general hospital. *Age and Ageing* **41**: 80–86.

Lapierre, S., Erlangsen, A., Waern, M. *et al.* (2011) Systematic review of elderly suicide prevention programs. *Crisis* **32**(2): 88–98.

Wilson, K., Mottram, P.G. & Vassilas, C. (2008) Psychotherapeutic treatments for older depressed people. *Cochrane Database of Systematic Reviews*, issue 1; CD004853. doi: 10.1002/14651858.

23 Dementia

Figure 23.1   The practice tree: Dementia

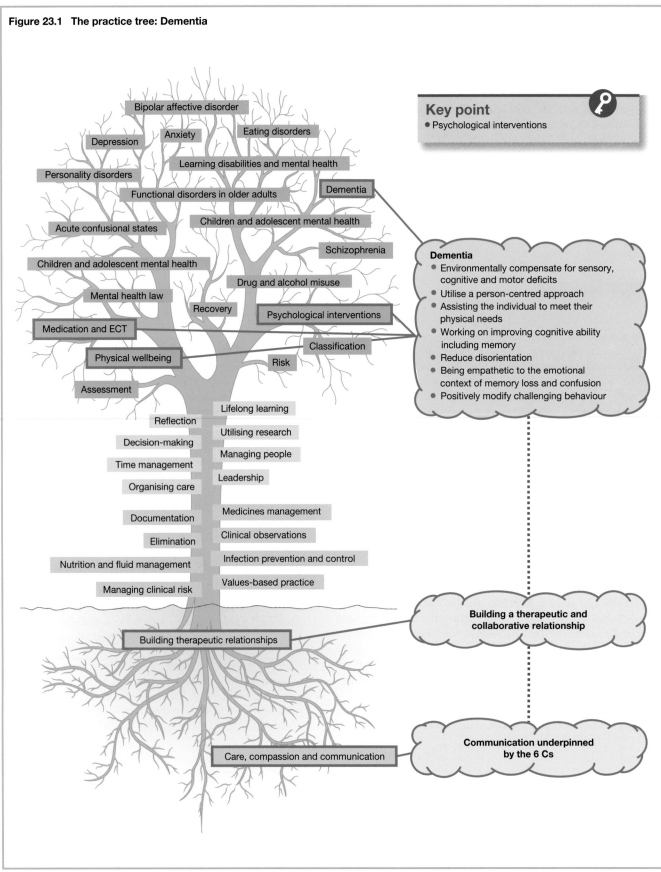

Key point
- Psychological interventions

Dementia
- Environmentally compensate for sensory, cognitive and motor deficits
- Utilise a person-centred approach
- Assisting the individual to meet their physical needs
- Working on improving cognitive ability including memory
- Reduce disorientation
- Being empathetic to the emotional context of memory loss and confusion
- Positively modify challenging behaviour

Building a therapeutic and collaborative relationship

Communication underpinned by the 6 Cs

Tree labels:
Bipolar affective disorder
Anxiety
Eating disorders
Depression
Learning disabilities and mental health
Personality disorders
Functional disorders in older adults
Dementia
Acute confusional states
Children and adolescent mental health
Children and adolescent mental health
Schizophrenia
Drug and alcohol misuse
Mental health law
Recovery
Psychological interventions
Medication and ECT
Classification
Physical wellbeing
Risk
Assessment
Lifelong learning
Reflection
Utilising research
Decision-making
Managing people
Time management
Leadership
Organising care
Documentation
Medicines management
Elimination
Clinical observations
Nutrition and fluid management
Infection prevention and control
Managing clinical risk
Values-based practice
Building therapeutic relationships
Care, compassion and communication

Mental Health Nursing at a Glance, First Edition. Grahame Smith. © 2015 John Wiley & Sons, Ltd. Published 2015 by John Wiley & Sons, Ltd.
Companion website: www.ataglanceseries.com/nursing/mentalhealth

Definitions

Dementia is viewed as a syndrome rather than a specific diagnosis. On this basis it is important to recognise there are different types of dementia with different causes and presentations. In DSM-5 dementia is now described as a major neurocognitive disorder (NCD). The dementias are organic disorders in that they result from an identified biological cause. The types of dementia include:
- Alzheimer's disease;
- vascular dementia;
- Parkinson 's disease;
- Dementia in Pick's disease;
- Dementia in Creutzfeldt–Jakob disease;
- Dementia in Huntington's disease;
- Dementia in human immunodeficiency virus infection;
- post-encephalitic dementia;
- head trauma-related dementia;
- alcohol-related dementia.

As a syndrome dementia is diagnosed when there are:
- multiple cognitive impairments including memory, orientation, language, comprehension and reasoning;
- a decline in social functioning;
- clear consciousness.

Clinical features

Dementia may present as a progressive decline in cognition and social functioning though it may also appear to have a sudden onset. The clinical features of the dementias include:
- apathy;
- aggression;
- restlessness;
- disinhibition;
- impulsivity;
- low mood;
- anxiety;
- delusion;
- hallucinations;
- sleep disturbances.

Risk factors

Dementia becomes more prevalent with age; the prevalence of dementia is less than 1% before the age of 65, increasing to 25% by the age of 90. Alzheimer's disease is the most common dementia, accounting for 55% of the dementias; vascular dementia accounts for about 25%. Besides age there are a number of other risk factors that may increase an individual's vulnerability:
- genetics;
- family history;
- Down's syndrome;
- cardiovascular problems;

- unhealthy diet;
- lack of physical activity;
- smoking.
- high levels of alcohol consumption;
- social isolation;
- head injury.

Management

Early diagnosis and early intervention in dementia are important especially where other mental disorders such as depression present a mixed clinical picture. This approach focuses on maintaining an individual's wellbeing. In terms of specific interventions treatment guidelines recommend:
- anti-dementia medication;
- cognitive stimulation;
- reality orientation therapy;
- validation therapy;
- behavioural therapy.

Psychological interventions

When nursing an individual diagnosed with a dementia it is important to consider that the environment has a significant role to play in keeping an individual well. Changes to an environment can compensate in part for reduced sensory, cognitive and motor ability. It is also important to ensure that an individual's physical needs are not neglected. Depending on the skill of the nurse the types of interventions (Figure 23.1) the nurse may deliver are:
- Establishing a therapeutic relationship based on a person-centred approach.
- Provide tailored support that focuses on assisting the individual to meet their physical needs.
- Working on improving cognitive ability including memory.
- Reducing disorientation through memory prompts both verbal and environmental.
- Being empathetic to the emotional context and meanings of someone experiencing memory loss and confusion.
- Provide behavioural strategies that positively modify challenging behaviour.

Further reading

Department of Health (2009) *Living Well with Dementia: A National Dementia Strategy*. London: Department of Health.

Moniz-Cook, E. & Manthorpe, J. (eds) (2009) *Early Psychological Interventions in Dementia: Evidence-Based Practice*. London: Jessica Kingsley.

National Institute for Clinical Excellence and Social Care Institute for Excellence (NICE-CIE) (2006) Dementia: Supporting People with Dementia and their Carers in Health and Social Care – NICE Clinical Guideline 42. London: NICE and SCIE.

24 Acute confusional states

Figure 24.1 The practice tree: Acute confusional states

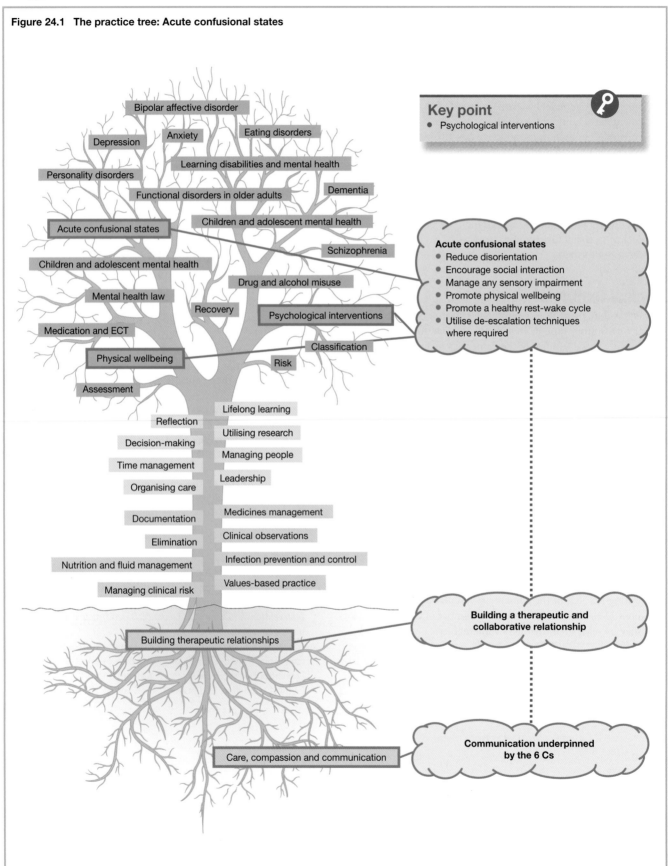

Key point
- Psychological interventions

Acute confusional states
- Reduce disorientation
- Encourage social interaction
- Manage any sensory impairment
- Promote physical wellbeing
- Promote a healthy rest-wake cycle
- Utilise de-escalation techniques where required

Bipolar affective disorder

Anxiety

Eating disorders

Depression

Personality disorders

Learning disabilities and mental health

Functional disorders in older adults

Dementia

Acute confusional states

Children and adolescent mental health

Children and adolescent mental health

Schizophrenia

Mental health law

Drug and alcohol misuse

Recovery

Psychological interventions

Medication and ECT

Physical wellbeing

Classification

Risk

Assessment

Lifelong learning

Reflection

Utilising research

Decision-making

Managing people

Time management

Leadership

Organising care

Documentation

Medicines management

Elimination

Clinical observations

Nutrition and fluid management

Infection prevention and control

Managing clinical risk

Values-based practice

Building therapeutic relationships

Building a therapeutic and collaborative relationship

Care, compassion and communication

Communication underpinned by the 6 Cs

Mental Health Nursing at a Glance, First Edition. Grahame Smith. © 2015 John Wiley & Sons, Ltd. Published 2015 by John Wiley & Sons, Ltd.
Companion website: www.ataglanceseries.com/nursing/mentalhealth

Definitions

An acute confusional state, or delirium, is characterised by severe confusion that has a rapid onset; the intensity of the symptoms can also fluctuate. There is usually a physical cause such as (Figure 24.2):

- alcohol, opiates, prescribed medication;
- renal, hepatic, cardiac failure;
- an underlying infection;
- hypoglycaemia;
- stroke;
- postoperative states.

Although delirium is viewed as a syndrome a diagnosis is made if the following are present:

- there is impaired consciousness and attention;
- perceptual or cognitive disturbances;
- sudden onset with fluctuating intensity;
- an identifiable cause.

Clinical features

As a clinical syndrome delirium can encompass a range of symptoms, which include:

- impaired consciousness and attention;
- memory problems;
- disorientation;
- language disturbances;
- hallucinations;
- transient delusions;
- sleep disturbances;
- drowsiness;
- fluctuating mood;
- restlessness;
- apathy;
- sweating;
- tachycardia.

Depending on the presentation of these symptoms delirium can be subdivided into three types:

- hypoactive delirium – quiet and withdrawn;
- hyperactive delirium – restless and agitated;
- mixed – features both types of behaviours.

Risk factors

Delirium can be difficult to diagnose as other conditions may resemble the symptoms of delirium, such as:

- depression;
- mania;
- dementia;
- schizophrenia.

Around one-third of older adults who are hospitalised present with delirium either on admission or during their hospital stay. There are a number of risk factors that may increase the risk of an individual developing the condition:

- age 65 or over ;
- diagnosed with a dementia;
- current hip fracture
- severe physical illness.

Management

The management of delirium focuses on the identification and treatment of the underlying cause. This entails carrying out a number of investigations, which may include:

- a full and comprehensive history;
- mental state assessment;

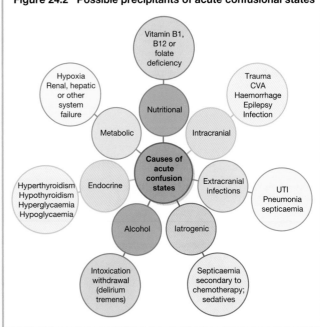

Figure 24.2 Possible precipitants of acute confusional states

- physical examination;
- blood tests;
- urine test;
- chest X-ray;
- brain imaging;
- electroencephalography (EEG).

Once the cause is identified then the underlying condition can be treated. Until the individual's acute confusional state is resolved treatment guidelines recommend the use of non-pharmacological interventions as a first option. Pharmacological interventions are recommended where distress and/or risk is not being sufficiently managed by the use of non-pharmacological interventions.

Psychological interventions

As delirium has an underlying physical cause most individuals with the condition will be nursed within an "adult nursing" environment such as an acute medical ward. When managing delirium (Figure 24.2) the mental health nurse will need to implement a series of preventative measures; these measures can also be used in the management of dementia:

- build a therapeutic relationship;
- reduce disorientation;
- promote physical wellbeing – nutrition and physical activity;
- utilise verbal and non-verbal de-escalation techniques where required.

Further reading

Royal College of Psychiatrists (2009) Factsheet: Delirium. London: Royal College of Psychiatrists Public Education Editorial Board.

Schofield, I. (2008) Delirium: challenges for clinical governance. *Journal of Nursing Management* **16**: 127–13.

Siddiqi, N., Young, J., House, A.O. *et al.* (2011) Stop Delirium! A complex intervention to prevent delirium in care homes: a mixed-methods feasibility study. *Age and Ageing* **40**: 90–98.

25 Drug and alcohol misuse

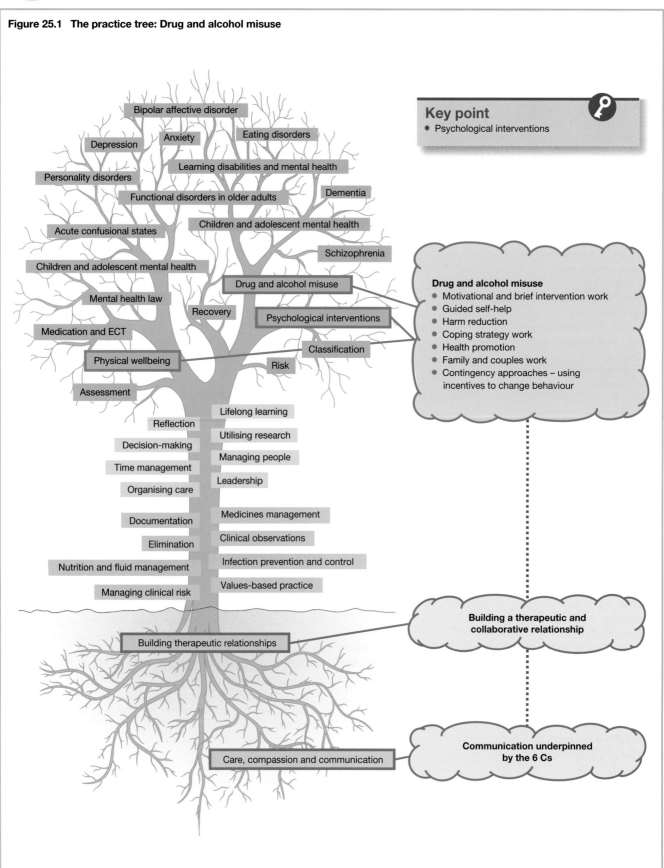

Figure 25.1 The practice tree: Drug and alcohol misuse

Bipolar affective disorder

Anxiety

Eating disorders

Depression

Learning disabilities and mental health

Personality disorders

Functional disorders in older adults

Dementia

Acute confusional states

Children and adolescent mental health

Children and adolescent mental health

Schizophrenia

Mental health law

Drug and alcohol misuse

Recovery

Psychological interventions

Medication and ECT

Classification

Physical wellbeing

Risk

Assessment

Lifelong learning

Reflection

Utilising research

Decision-making

Managing people

Time management

Leadership

Organising care

Documentation

Medicines management

Elimination

Clinical observations

Nutrition and fluid management

Infection prevention and control

Managing clinical risk

Values-based practice

Building therapeutic relationships

Care, compassion and communication

Key point
- Psychological interventions

Drug and alcohol misuse
- Motivational and brief intervention work
- Guided self-help
- Harm reduction
- Coping strategy work
- Health promotion
- Family and couples work
- Contingency approaches – using incentives to change behaviour

Building a therapeutic and collaborative relationship

Communication underpinned by the 6 Cs

Definitions

Drug and alcohol misuse is where an individual's drug and/or alcohol use has a harmful impact, which can relate to physical, social and psychological harms. The individual may or may not be dependent on the drug/s or alcohol; signs of dependency include:

- compulsion to take the drug or alcohol;
- adverse impact upon the individual's social functioning;
- tolerant to the drug or alcohol;
- the individual has difficulty in controlling their drug or alcohol use;
- stopping their drug or alcohol use can cause withdrawal symptoms.

Generally illicit drugs can be divided into:

- opiates;
- stimulants;
- hallucinogens;
- cannabis.

Alcohol use is usually described in terms of safe limits; 21 units of alcohol per week for men and 14 units for women (a unit of alcohol is approximately a small glass of wine or half pint of beer). Alcohol abuse can be divided into:

- Hazardous drinking – men consume between 22 and 50 units and women between 15 and 35 units weekly.
- Harmful drinking – men consume over 50 units and women over 35 units weekly.
- Binge drinking – consuming double the safe limit of units in one day.

Drug and alcohol disorders include:

- acute intoxication;
- harmful use;
- dependence;
- withdrawal state;
- psychotic disorder;
- amnesic disorder.

Clinical features

The effect of a substance depends on the type of drug; opiates can cause drowsiness whereas stimulants can cause restlessness. Generally substance misuse can lead to:

- disturbances of consciousness and perception;
- damage to an individual's health and social functioning;
- neglect;
- physical and psychological withdrawal;
- hallucinations and delusions;
- memory and cognitive impairments.

Risk factors

It is estimated in the UK that one in ten adults have used an illicit substance: cannabis is the most commonly used drug. In terms of alcohol consumption around a quarter of the population exceeds the safe limits. The causes of substance misuse are not clear though there are risk factors that may increase an individual's vulnerability:

- availability of the substance;
- peer pressure;
- a comorbid mental health disorder;
- stressful situations or circumstances;
- family history;
- life events – childhood abuse and loss.

Management

The management of substance misuse is dependent on the presentation, an individual can present with signs of acute intoxication, withdrawal or dependency. The assessment of the individual is extremely important as a head injury can present as acute intoxication especially where an individual has also been drinking. In terms of specific interventions treatment guidelines recommend:

- acute detoxification;
- motivational enhancement therapy;
- cognitive behaviour therapy;
- abstinence;
- social learning strategies;
- harm reduction strategies;
- self-help groups;
- medication – manage cravings.

Psychological interventions

It is important to note that an individual's substance use can change over time. This may include stopping their alcohol or drug misuse. Individuals who misuse substances and access services are usually treated outside the mental health in-patient setting, though mental health nurses within this type of setting will encounter individuals who both misuse substances and have a comorbid mental health disorder. As the mental health nurse will work in a variety of settings they may after the detoxification phase need to deliver different types of psychological interventions (Figure 25.1), which include:

- build a collaborative and therapeutic relationship;
- motivational and brief intervention work;
- guided self-help;
- harm reduction;
- coping strategy work;
- health promotion;
- family and couples work;
- contingency approaches – using incentives to change behaviour.

Further reading

National Institute for Health and Clinical Excellence (NICE) (2007) *Drug Misuse Psychosocial Interventions – NICE Clinical Guideline 51*. London: NICE.

National Institute for Health and Clinical Excellence (NICE) (2011) *Alcohol-use Disorders, Diagnosis, Assessment and Management of Harmful Drinking and Alcohol Dependence – NICE Clinical Guideline 115*. London: NICE.

Miller, W.R. & Rollnick, S. (1991) *Motivational Interviewing: Preparing People to Change Addictive Behaviour*. London: Guilford Press.

26 Children and adolescent mental health

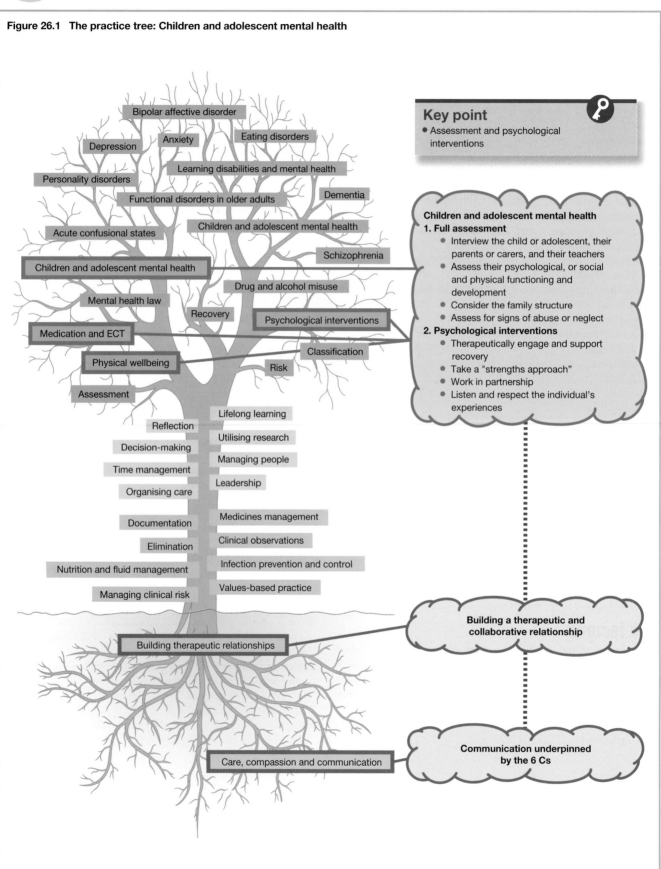

Figure 26.1 The practice tree: Children and adolescent mental health

Bipolar affective disorder

Anxiety

Eating disorders

Depression

Learning disabilities and mental health

Personality disorders

Functional disorders in older adults

Dementia

Children and adolescent mental health

Acute confusional states

Schizophrenia

Children and adolescent mental health

Drug and alcohol misuse

Mental health law

Recovery

Psychological interventions

Medication and ECT

Classification

Physical wellbeing

Risk

Assessment

Lifelong learning

Reflection

Utilising research

Decision-making

Managing people

Time management

Leadership

Organising care

Documentation

Medicines management

Elimination

Clinical observations

Nutrition and fluid management

Infection prevention and control

Managing clinical risk

Values-based practice

Building therapeutic relationships

Care, compassion and communication

Key point
- Assessment and psychological interventions

Children and adolescent mental health
1. Full assessment
- Interview the child or adolescent, their parents or carers, and their teachers
- Assess their psychological, or social and physical functioning and development
- Consider the family structure
- Assess for signs of abuse or neglect

2. Psychological interventions
- Therapeutically engage and support recovery
- Take a "strengths approach"
- Work in partnership
- Listen and respect the individual's experiences

Building a therapeutic and collaborative relationship

Communication underpinned by the 6 Cs

Definitions

Mental health problems in children and adolescents can be mild to severe; some problems may last for a short period of time, and others may last a lot longer. They have a tendency to interfere with a child's or an adolescent's normal development, which includes their ability to function socially and/or psychologically. Specific childhood disorders include:
- hyperkinetic disorders;
- conduct disorders;
- emotional disorders;
- social functioning disorders;
- other disorders – enuresis, encopresis;
- pervasive development disorders (Autism Spectrum Disorder – DSM-5).

There are also mental disorders that can start in childhood, including:
- depression;
- anxiety disorders;
- adjustment disorders;
- psychotic disorders;
- sleep problems.
   Disorders in adolescence include:
- conduct disorder;
- eating disorders;
- mood disorders;
- anxiety disorders;
- obsessive-compulsive disorder;
- schizophrenia;
- substance misuse.

Though not a disorder, self-harm is common in adolescence. It is reported that 1 in 12 adolescents self-harm, with overdosing on paracetamol being the most common known method.

Clinical features

Mental health problems in children and adolescents according to age can present in different ways. For example, separation anxiety is common in younger children who worry about being separated from their parents or carers. Normally this fear subsides but for other children it can persist or reappear in adolescence, where it has an adverse impact upon their ability to function. On this basis it is important that a full assessment (see Figure 26.1) is carried out, which includes:
- Interviewing the child or adolescent, their parents or carers, and their teachers.
- Assessing the child's or adolescent's psychological, social and physical functioning and development.
- Considering the family structure.
- Assessing for signs of abuse or neglect.

Risk factors

The prevalence of mental health disorders in children and adolescents is between 10 and 20%, with boys having a higher prevalence than girls. The causes of these mental health problems are not clear though there are risk factors that may increase an individual's vulnerability:
- comorbid genetic disorder;
- physical health problems;
- poor educational performance;
- a comorbid mental health disorder;
- family difficulties;
- overprotective parents;
- parents with a mental health problem;
- stress, trauma;
- abuse or neglect;
- bullying;
- loss.

Management

The management of mental health problems in children and adolescents is dependent on the presentation and also the level of complexity. On this basis children and adolescent mental health services are designed around a tier system:
- Tier 1 – interventions provided by practitioners who are not mental health specialists working in universal services.
- Tier 2 – interventions provided by mental health practitioners working in community or primary care teams.
- Tier 3 – interventions provided by mental health teams for children and adolescents with severe, complex and persistent mental health needs.
- Tier 4 – similar to tier 3 but there is a higher level of risk identified.
   In terms of specific interventions treatment guidelines recommend:
- cognitive behaviour therapy;
- family therapy;
- group and individual therapy;
- solution-focused therapy.

Psychological interventions

When working with children and adolescents with mental health problems the mental health nurse needs to be competent in delivering the required interventions. The nurse may in some cases be supervised by a specialist in this area or they may be required to follow an agreed plan of care (Figure 26.1), which may include:
- therapeutically engage and support recovery;
- take a "strengths approach";
- work in partnership;
- listen and respect the individual's experiences.

Further reading

National Institute for Clinical Excellence (NICE) (2005) Depression in Children and Young People: Identification and Management in Primary, Community and Secondary Care – Clinical Guideline 28. London: NICE.

National Institute for Health and Clinical Excellence (NICE) (2008) Attention Deficit Hyperactivity Disorder: Diagnosis and Management of ADHD in Children, Young People and Adults – Clinical Guideline 72. London: NICE.

Rober, P. (2008) Being there, experiencing and creating space for dialogue: about working with children in family therapy. *Journal of Family Therapy* **30**: 465–77.

27 Recovery

Figure 27.1   The practice tree: Recovery

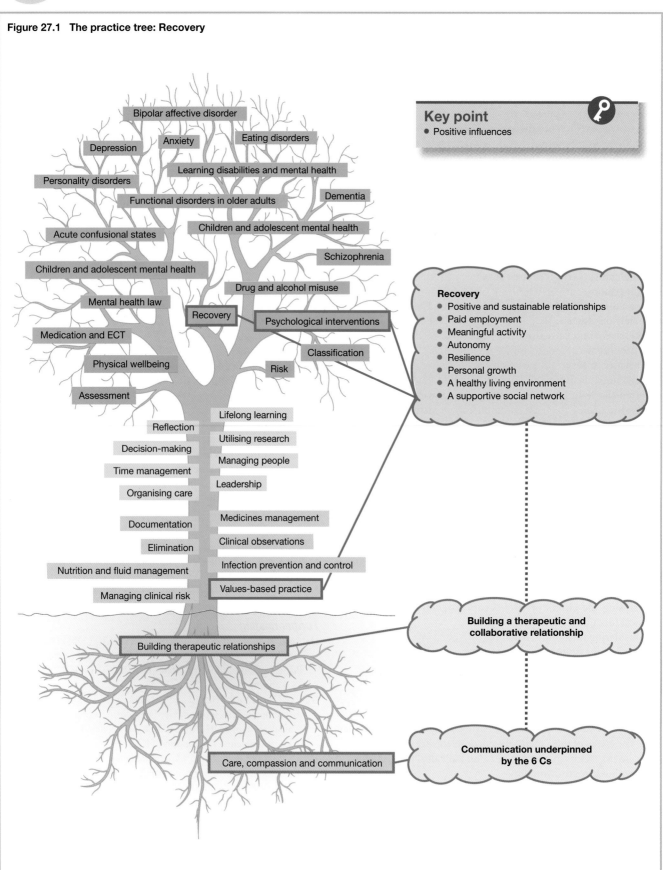

Key point
- Positive influences

Recovery
- Positive and sustainable relationships
- Paid employment
- Meaningful activity
- Autonomy
- Resilience
- Personal growth
- A healthy living environment
- A supportive social network

Building a therapeutic and collaborative relationship

Communication underpinned by the 6 Cs

Mental Health Nursing at a Glance, First Edition. Grahame Smith. © 2015 John Wiley & Sons, Ltd. Published 2015 by John Wiley & Sons, Ltd.
Companion website: www.ataglanceseries.com/nursing/mentalhealth

Introduction

Recovery as a therapeutic process is an integral part of mental health nursing practice. As a process mental health nurses often see recovery in terms of eliminating or controlling symptoms of mental distress. This view is quite a narrow, as recovery should be a whole-person approach where the meaning of recovery is embedded within the hopes and aspirations of the individual. Recovery is also about social inclusion where individuals are supported to live meaningful lives within society.

Competencies

Mental health nurses are required to:
- Effectively engage with individuals with mental health problems in a way that is person-centred and also promotes social inclusion and recovery.
- Ensure their practice is recovery-focused whatever the context or setting and that it values, respects and explores the meaning of an individual's mental distress.
- Promote the self-determination and expertise of individuals with mental health problems while using their personal qualities and interpersonal skills to develop and maintain a recovery-focused therapeutic relationship.
- Work with people living with mental distress, other professionals and agencies to shape services in a way that aids recovery.

The context

Utilising a recovery-based approach presents a significant challenge for mental health nurses especially where there are professional and policy drivers for such an approach but no single agreed definition of recovery. On this basis recovery should be seen as being relative to the individual and their circumstances, meaning that the recovery process for that individual is being constantly redefined by their ever-changing needs. The challenge for the mental health nurse in these circumstances is that they need to be both receptive and responsive to the service user's ever-evolving needs in a way that their practice is positively redefined by these experiences. Even though recovery as process is relative in nature it can be seen to have aims that include:
- promoting wellbeing;
- maximising opportunity;
- empowering individuals to take control;
- facilitating and supporting the individual in finding meaning and purpose.

The recovery process

Recovery can also be described in terms of a process that includes the following features:
- A whole-person approach is taken rather than just focusing on symptoms.
- Recovery is viewed as a "journey rather than a destination".
- Optimism, commitment and hope are key values.
- Support should be systematic but also innovative.

The components of recovery

There are a number of "models" of recovery such as the:
- collaborative recovery model;
- strengths model;
- tidal model;
- wellbeing and recovery action plan approach.

The tidal model is particularly pertinent to mental health nurses as it has been created by mental health nurses in collaboration with mental health service users. As an approach the tidal model is made up of three key components or domains:
- Self-domain – narrative or story-telling component.
- World domain – where this narrative component is shared with others.
- Others domain – this is where recovery is enacted through the care delivery process.

The recovery approach

The mental health nurse in the recovery process must be able to support the individual in a way that the individual's story is actively valued as a core part of the care delivery process. The nurse must also recognise that interventions have to be outcome focused but they also have to be adaptable to changing need. Building on this the nurse must also be aware of the factors (Figure 27.1) that positively influence the recovery process; these include:
- positive and sustainable relationships;
- paid employment;
- meaningful activity;
- autonomy;
- resilience;
- personal growth;
- a healthy living environment;
- a supportive social network.

Further reading

Barker, P.J. & Buchanan-Barker, P. (2005) *The Tidal Model: A Guide for Mental Health Professionals*. London: Brunner-Routledge.

Copeland, M.E. (1997) *Wellness Recovery Action Plan*. Dummerston: Peach Press.

Mackeith, J. & Burns, S. (2008) *Mental Health Recovery Star: User Guide*. London: Mental Health Providers' Forum and Triangle Consulting.

28 # Physical wellbeing

Figure 28.1 The practice tree: Physical wellbeing

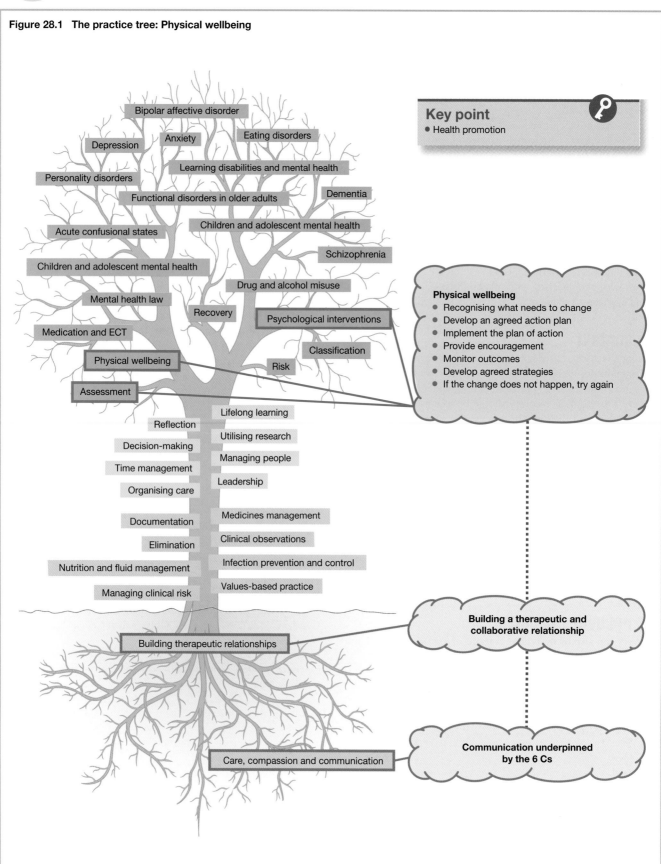

Key point
- Health promotion

Physical wellbeing
- Recognising what needs to change
- Develop an agreed action plan
- Implement the plan of action
- Provide encouragement
- Monitor outcomes
- Develop agreed strategies
- If the change does not happen, try again

Bipolar affective disorder
Depression
Anxiety
Eating disorders
Learning disabilities and mental health
Personality disorders
Functional disorders in older adults
Dementia
Acute confusional states
Children and adolescent mental health
Schizophrenia
Children and adolescent mental health
Drug and alcohol misuse
Mental health law
Recovery
Psychological interventions
Medication and ECT
Classification
Physical wellbeing
Risk
Assessment
Lifelong learning
Reflection
Utilising research
Decision-making
Managing people
Time management
Leadership
Organising care
Documentation
Medicines management
Elimination
Clinical observations
Nutrition and fluid management
Infection prevention and control
Managing clinical risk
Values-based practice

Building therapeutic relationships

Building a therapeutic and collaborative relationship

Care, compassion and communication

Communication underpinned by the 6 Cs

Mental Health Nursing at a Glance, First Edition. Grahame Smith. © 2015 John Wiley & Sons, Ltd. Published 2015 by John Wiley & Sons, Ltd.
Companion website: www.ataglanceseries.com/nursing/mentalhealth

Introduction

The role of the mental health nurse is to promote good physical health and wellbeing. This is especially important when considering that individuals diagnosed with a severe mental health problem are more likely to experience physical health problems than the general population. The first stage of promoting good physical health and wellbeing is to ensure that an individual's physical health needs are identified. This process should take the form of regular physical assessments; any needs identified should be addressed through an integrated and holistic package of care. Mental health nurses will also be required to deliver physical health care and/or signpost individuals to the appropriate services (Figure 28.1).

Competencies

Mental health nurses are required to:
• promote physical health and wellbeing through education, role modelling and effective communication;
• deliver physical care that meets the essential needs of people with mental health problems;
• recognise and respond to the physical needs of all individuals who come into their care;
• be able where required to signpost an individual with physical and mental health problems to the appropriate service.

The context

Physical health problems are common in individuals diagnosed with severe mental illness, such as depression, schizophrenia and bipolar affective disorder. The types of physical health problems include:
• cardiovascular disease;
• respiratory problems;
• diabetes;
• digestive disorders;
• obesity;
• musculoskeletal diseases;
• cancer – lung, colorectal and breast cancer;
• viral infections.
It is also important to recognise that physical ill health can lead to a mental health problem. It is not uncommon for enduring physical health problems to be comorbid with depression; these include:
• cancer;
• heart disease;
• diabetes;
• musculoskeletal problems;
• respiratory problems.

Factors

There are numerous factors that may account for a higher incidence of physical ill health in individuals with mental health problems. These factors include:
• Psychiatric medication – some medications increase the risk of obesity, diabetes and cardiac problems.

• Lifestyle – individuals with mental health problems have a higher rate of smoking, and drug and alcohol misuse; they also tend to eat less well, and exercise less.
• Social – indirect factors such as poverty, poor housing, and unemployment may also have an adverse impact.
   There are also protective factors that keep mental health service users physically well, such as:
• supportive and nurturing social networks;
• employment;
• self-awareness and having a sense of hope;
• having a healthy lifestyle.

Physical health assessment

Even when these factors are taken into account, individuals with mental health problems are less likely to have their physical health needs recognised compared to the general population. On this basis a physical health assessment should include:
• the gathering of baseline physical health data including a medical history;
• a physical examination including baseline observations;
• baseline investigations including blood tests.
After the initial assessment the individual should be monitored annually, usually by their general practitioner.

Managing physical health

The mental health nurse's role in managing an individual's physical health is to be a health promoter; this includes:
• providing education about medication and its side-effects;
• providing dietary advice or signpost to a dietician;
• promoting the benefits of physical exercise and monitoring weight;
• providing smoking cessation advice;
• liaising with the GP where required;
• signpost to family planning and sexual health services where required.
   A key part of health promotion is to work collaboratively with the individual to change unhealthy behaviours by:
• recognising what behaviour needs to change;
• developing an agreed action plan;
• implementing the plan of action;
• providing encouragement however small the change;
• monitoring outcomes;
• developing agreed strategies that maintain change;
• if the change does not happen, try again.

Further reading

Department of Health (2011) *No Health Without Mental Health: A Cross-Government Mental Health Outcomes Strategy for People of All Ages*. London: HMG/Department of Health.
New Economics Foundation (2008) *Five Ways to Well-being: The Evidence*. London: New Economics Foundation.
McManus, S., Meltzer, H. & Brugha, T. (2009) *Adult Psychiatric Morbidity in England, 2007: Results of a Household Survey*. Leeds: NHS Information Centre for Health and Social Care.

29 Mental health law

Figure 29.1   The practice tree: Mental health law

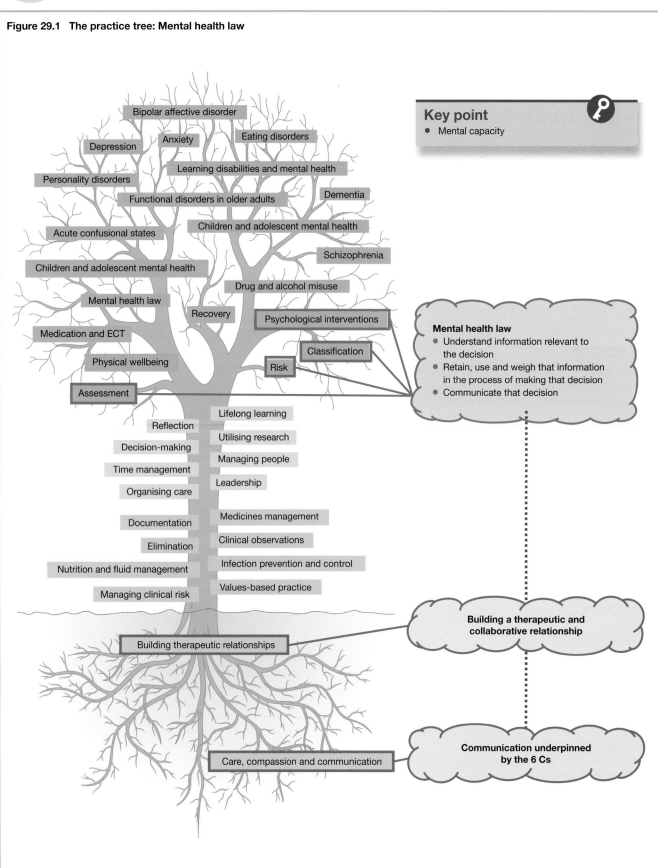

Introduction

Mental health nurses on a day-to-day basis have to make practice decisions that must be consistent with a number of legal frameworks. The added dimension in mental health nursing is that these decisions may relate to either restricting a mental health service user's freedoms or, where these restrictions are in place, maintaining the use of these restrictions. This does not mean that a mental health user does not have rights – it is quite the opposite – and on this basis it is important that the mental health nurse knows how to balance autonomy against managing risk.

Competencies

Mental health nurses are required to:
• Understand and apply current legislation in a way that protects vulnerable individuals within their practice.
• Act within the law when collaboratively working with individuals living with mental health problems.
• Respect and uphold a mental health service user's rights in accordance with the law and relevant ethical and regulatory frameworks including taking into account local protocols.
• Know when to actively share personal information with others when the interests of safety and protection override the need for confidentiality.

The context

There are a number of legal frameworks that mental health nurses need to understand and work within. Not all of these frameworks are specific to mental health care (e.g. the Human Rights Act); nonetheless the mental health nurse must still be able to work with and understand these frameworks. In relation to what is called mental health law, such as the Mental Health Act 1983 for England and Wales, the mental health nurse will work within a framework that allows them in certain circumstance to restrict freedoms. They will also work with legal frameworks that support individuals with severe mental problems to make decisions; such frameworks include the Mental Capacity Act 2005, applying to England and Wales.

The Human Rights Act

The Human Rights Act 1998 came into full force in the UK in 2000. The Act protects the rights of the individual through a number of Articles. All these Articles are relevant to individuals with mental health problems but where an individual's freedoms are restricted the following Articles have particular relevance:
• the right to life (Article 2);
• the prohibition of torture (Article 3);
• the right to liberty and security (Article 5);
• the right to respect for private and family life (Article 8).

The Mental Capacity Act

Generally individuals are presumed to have the capacity (Figure 29.2) to make their own decisions, such as:
• understand information relevant to the decision;
• retain, use and weigh that information in the process of making that decision;
• communicate that decision.

Where individuals lack capacity there is a supportive and transparent process enshrined within the Mental Capacity Act 2005. This process acknowledges that a lack of capacity may be temporary and transient and that individuals lacking capacity should where possible be helped to make their decisions (Figure 29.2). This Act applies to England and Wales; Scotland has similar legislation, the Adults with Incapacity Act 2000. Northern Ireland does not have specific legislation but relevant legislation includes the Enduring Powers of Attorney Order 1987.

Figure 29.2 What does the Mental Capacity Act (2005) (England and Wales) do?

Gives any adult with capacity the right to make:
Advance decision(s)
Lasting Power of Attorney

And

Says how to decide if someone has capacity

And

For any adult without capacity it tells professionals to:

Act in their best interests	Apply Deprivation of Liberty
Consult family/ friends about decisions	Safeguards (DoLS)
Appoint Independent Mental Capacity	to anyone deprived of liberty
Advocate (IMCA) for important decisions	

Souce: Katona et al. (2012) Psychiatry at a Glance, 5th edn. Reproduced with permission of Wiley.

Table 29.1 Summary of main civil (not forensic) sections of the Mental Health Act (MHA)

MHA Section	Purpose	Recommendations	Application†	Duration
2	Assessment	2 doctors	AMHP[a] or nearest relative (NR)	20 days
3	Treatment	2 doctors	AMHP or NR	6 months
Community Treatment Order	Treatment in community of patient previously detained on Section 3 or 37		Responsible clinician (agreed with AMHP)	6 months
4	Urgent assessment from community (no time to arrange Section 2)	1 doctors (AC)	AMHP or NR	72 hours
5(2)	Urgent detention of inpatient	1 doctor		72 hours
5(4)	Urgent detention of psychiatric inpatient in absence of doctor	Registered mental nurse		6 hours
135	Removal from home to place of safety	Police officer		72 hours
136	Removal from public place to place of safety	Police officer		72 hours

[a] AMHP, Approved Mental Health Professional.

Source: Katona et al. (2012) Psychiatry at a Glance, 5th edn. Reproduced with permission of Wiley

Table 29.2 Summary of main forensic sections of the Mental Health Act

Section	What does it do?	Recommendations	Who applies	Length
35	Remands an accused person to hospital for a report	1 doctor	Crown or Magistrates' Court	28 days
36	Remands an accused person to hospital for treatment Appropriate medical treatment must be available	2 doctors (1 approved)	Crown Court	28 days
37	Orders a hospital admission or guardianship of a person convicted of an imprisonable offence (except murder)	2 doctors	Crown or Magistrates' Court	6 months
38	Sends convicted person to hospital for treatment prior to sentencing	2 doctors	Crown or Magistrates' Court	28 days
41	Applies restriction that patient on another hospital section may not be given leave, transferred or discharged, without the Home Secretary's consent	1 doctor	Crown Court	Duration of other section
47	Transfers sentenced prisoner to hospital for treatment	2 doctors	Home Office	6 months

Source: Katona et al. (2012) Psychiatry at a Glance, 5th edn. Reproduced with permission of Wiley

Table 29.3 Provisions of the Mental Health Act for treatment without consent

Section	Type of treatment	What it says
2 and 3 (and equivalent forensic sections)	Medication for first three months	May be given without consent
56	Medication on sections 2 and 3 after three months ECT at any time	/Patient must consent (and be attested competent to do so by the RC[a]) **OR** an independent **Second Approved Doctor (SOAD)** nominated by the MHAC[b] must: • Interview the patient • Discuss the treatment wth the RC and two other professionals involved in the patient's treatment • Agree the treatment is necessary ECT cannot be given to patients with capacity without their consent
57	Psychosurgery Surgical hormone implants	Needs both c onsent and a second opinion
62	Life-savine treatment	Exempt from Sections 57 and 58

[a] RC, **Responsible Clinician.**
[b] **MHAC**, Mental Health Act Commission.

Source: Katona et al. (2012) Psychiatry at a Glance, 5th edn. Reproduced with permission of Wiley

Table 29.4 The main compulsory orders under the Mental Health (Care and Treatment) (Scotland) Act 2003

MHA order	Purpose	Location	Requirements	Maximum duration
Emergency detention	Detention for urgent assessment if arranging short-term detention order would involve undesirable delay	Hospital	Certification by any fully registered doctor Agreement of an MHO[a] if possible	72 hours
Short-term detention	Assessment or treatment	Hospital or community	Recmmendation by two AMP[b] Application by MHO Decision by Mental Health Review Tribunal	6 months

[a] AMP, Approved Medical Practitioner.
[b] MHO, Mental Health Officer.

Source: Katona et al. (2012) Psychiatry at a Glance, 5th edn. Reproduced with permission of Wiley

Table 29.5 The main assessment and treatment orders under the Mental Health (Care and Treatment) (Scotland) Act 2003

MHA order	Purpose	Location	Requirements	Maximum duration
Assessment	Assessment	Hospital	Made by court Evidence from one doctor	28 days
Interim compulson	Longer period of assessment	Hospital	Made by court Evidence from two doctors (one an AMP)	1 year (renewal every 12 weeks)
Treatment	Treatment	Hospital	Made by court Evidence from two doctors (one an AMP)	Until end of remand period or sentence
Compulsion	Similar to a CTO[a] (see above), except the requirement for significantly impaired decision-making ability with regard to treatment does not apply	Hospital	Made by court Evidence from two doctors (one an AMP) Report from the desigated MHO	6 months
Restriction	Any change in the legal statusof the patient must be referred to Scottish Ministers and the Tribunal	Hospital		Added to compulsion
Transfer for treatment directions	Transfer of prisoners to hospitalfor mental health treatment	Hospital	Made by Scottish ministers Evidence from two doctors (one in AMP)	Until sentence expires)

[a]CTO, Compulsory Treatment Order.
Source: Katona et al. (2012) Psychiatry at a Glance, 5th edn. Reproduced with permission of Wiley

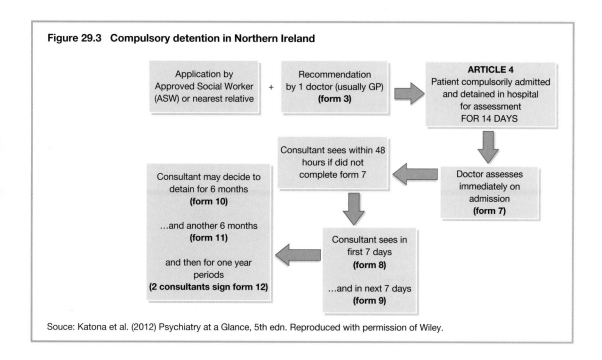

Figure 29.3 Compulsory detention in Northern Ireland

Souce: Katona et al. (2012) Psychiatry at a Glance, 5th edn. Reproduced with permission of Wiley.

Further reading

Jones, R. (2013) Mental Health Act Manual, 16th edn. London: Sweet & Maxwell.
Mental Health Law Online. URL: http://www.mentalhealthlaw.co.uk/Main_Page
Mind. Mental health legislation news. URL: http://www.mind.org.uk/news?gclid=COCA9Nnkk7kCFSXLtAodDVoAoA

The Mental Health Act

The Mental Health Act (MHA) 1983 of England and Wales amended by the MHA 2007 is the legal framework under which an individual can be compulsory admitted, detained and treated in hospital. There is also a Community Treatment Order (CTO) where an individual following discharge from either a Section 3 or Section 37 may be recalled back to hospital on certain grounds.

Summary tables of the main civil and forensic sections (Tables 29.1 and 29.2).

Some of these sections under certain circumstances allow an individual with a mental health problem to be treated without their consent (Table 29.3).

Scotland has similar legislation, the Mental Health Act 2003; see the main compulsory orders and the main assessment and treatment orders (Tables 29.4 and 29.5).

In the case of Northern Ireland the 1986 Mental Health Order is still in effect; it is planned that it will be replaced by the Mental Capacity Bill in 2013/14 (Fig 29.3).

The use of these legal frameworks are monitored by the Mental Act Commission in England and Wales, the Mental Welfare Commission in Scotland, and in Northern Ireland the Mental Health Commission.

30 Medication and ECT

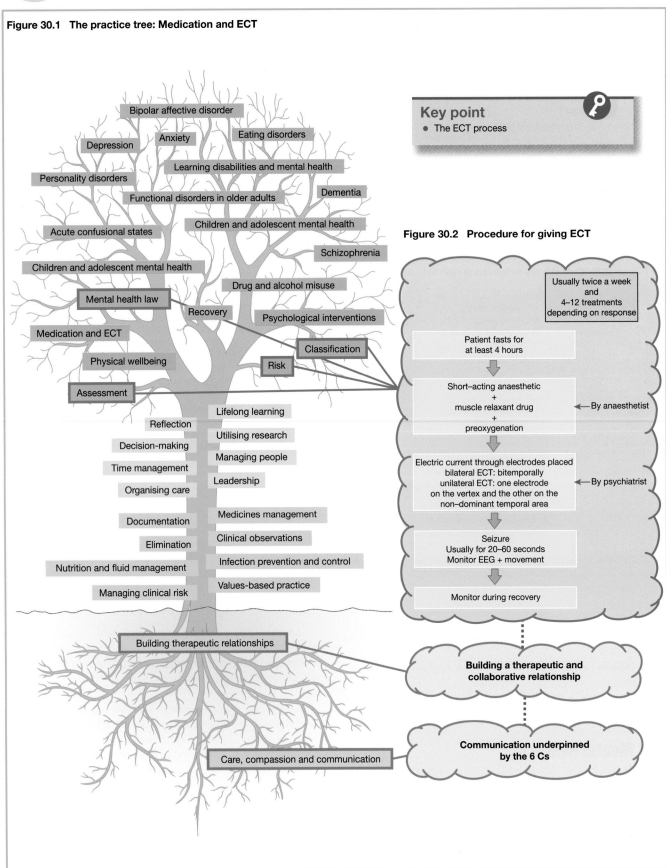

Figure 30.1   The practice tree: Medication and ECT

Bipolar affective disorder

Anxiety

Eating disorders

Depression

Personality disorders

Learning disabilities and mental health

Functional disorders in older adults

Dementia

Acute confusional states

Children and adolescent mental health

Schizophrenia

Children and adolescent mental health

Drug and alcohol misuse

Mental health law

Recovery

Psychological interventions

Medication and ECT

Classification

Physical wellbeing

Risk

Assessment

Lifelong learning

Reflection

Utilising research

Decision-making

Managing people

Time management

Leadership

Organising care

Documentation

Medicines management

Elimination

Clinical observations

Nutrition and fluid management

Infection prevention and control

Managing clinical risk

Values-based practice

Building therapeutic relationships

Care, compassion and communication

Key point
● The ECT process

Figure 30.2   Procedure for giving ECT

Usually twice a week
and
4–12 treatments
depending on response

Patient fasts for
at least 4 hours

Short–acting anaesthetic
+
muscle relaxant drug
+
preoxygenation
← By anaesthetist

Electric current through electrodes placed
bilateral ECT: bitemporally
unilateral ECT: one electrode
on the vertex and the other on the
non–dominant temporal area
← By psychiatrist

Seizure
Usually for 20–60 seconds
Monitor EEG + movement

Monitor during recovery

Building a therapeutic and
collaborative relationship

Communication underpinned
by the 6 Cs

Introduction

Mental health nurses when working with a mental health service user will deliver a number of nursing interventions; it is not unusual for the administration of psychiatric medication to be one of these interventions. On this basis it is important for the mental health nurse not only to understand what they are administrating, but also to know how medication fits with the other interventions that they provide. The nurse also needs to an educator, which means being able to provide information to individuals with mental health problems about the medication they have been prescribed. In some cases a mental health service user may be receiving electroconvulsive therapy (ECT); in this situation the mental health nurse would take a similar approach.

Competencies

Mental health nurses are required to:
- Ensure that they have an in-depth knowledge of common mental health treatments.
- Offer holistic care and, working as part of the multi-professional team, offer a range of treatment options of which medicines may form a part.
- Assist individuals with mental health problems to make informed choices about pharmacological and physical treatments they may receive.
- Provide education, information and support related to the provision of pharmacological and physical treatments.

The context

Psychiatric medication started to become available during the latter part of the 19th century. Though it was not until the 1950s that medication used in psychiatry was seen as a viable treatment option. Psychiatric medication can be described as a licensed medication that exerts a desired effect on the brain and nervous system. These medications can be prescribed for a range of mental disorders; they usually form part of a package of care that would also include psychological approaches. Electroconvulsive therapy (ECT) is a treatment administered under a short-acting anaesthetic in which seizures are electrically induced. Usually ECT is prescribed for use as a treatment for severe depression that has not responded to other treatments.

ECT

ECT is indicated in the case of:
- severe depression;
- a severe and prolonged episode of mania that has not responded to treatment;
- moderate depression that has not responded to multiple drug treatments.

Cognitive impairment can be a side-effect of treatment. The procedure for giving ECT is shown in Figure 30.2.

Types of psychiatric medication

The main groups of psychiatric medication are:
- antidepressants;
- antipsychotics;
- anxiolytics and hypnotics;
- mood stabilisers;
- antidementia drugs.

Antipsychotics

Antipsychotics are used to treat the symptoms of psychosis such as delusions, hallucinations and thought disorder. It is thought that they reduce the symptoms of psychosis by blocking the dopamine (D2/3) receptors in the brain. There are two categories of antipsychotics, the typical antipsychotics and the atypical antipsychotics (Figure 30.3). Both categories of antipsychotics have a number of side-effects, which include movement disorders, sedation and weight gain (Figure 30.4).

30 Medication and ECT - ctd
Antidepressants

Antidepressants are used to treat depression, usually moderate to severe depression. It is thought they work by increasing the transmission of the monoamines (serotonin, noradrenaline and occasionally dopamine) in the brain. There are a number of categories of antidepressants and different categories may cause different side-effects (Figure 30.5).

Anxiolytics and hypnotics

Benzodiazepines are the most common category of drugs in this group. They are effective for the short-term treatment of generalised anxiety, insomnia, alcohol withdrawal states, and the control of violent behaviour. They work by potentiating the inhibitory effects of gamma-aminobutyric acid in the brain; on this basis they induce sleep and muscle relaxation. Zopiclone and zolpidem are hypnotics; they have a similar action to the benzodiazepines but without the muscle relaxation. Another drug, buspirone, is used in the short-term treatment of anxiety.

Mood stabilisers

Lithium is used in the treatment of recurrent bipolar affective disorder; its mechanism of action is unknown. It can be toxic above a certain serum concentration range; the optimal range is 0.4–1.0 mmol/L. Monitoring of the drug should include thyroid and renal function tests before commencement of the drug and

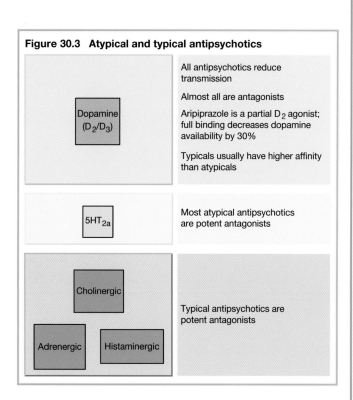

Figure 30.3 Atypical and typical antipsychotics

Dopamine (D$_2$/D$_3$)

All antipsychotics reduce transmission

Almost all are antagonists

Aripiprazole is a partial D$_2$ agonist; full binding decreases dopamine availability by 30%

Typicals usually have higher affinity than atypicals

5HT$_{2a}$

Most atypical antipsychotics are potent antagonists

Cholinergic

Adrenergic

Histaminergic

Typical antipsychotics are potent antagonists

Figure 30.4 Side-effects of antipsychotics

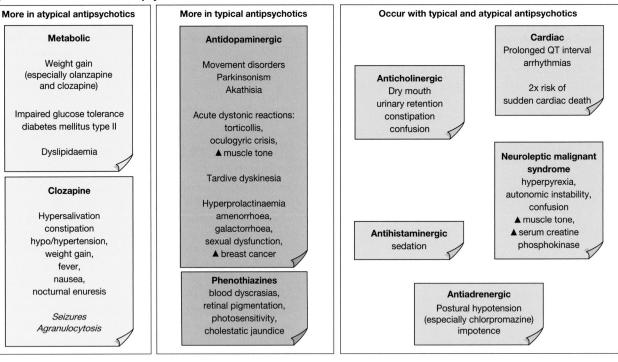

More in atypical antipsychotics	More in typical antipsychotics	Occur with typical and atypical antipsychotics
Metabolic Weight gain (especially olanzapine and clozapine) Impaired glucose tolerance diabetes mellitus type II Dyslipidaemia	**Antidopaminergic** Movement disorders Parkinsonism Akathisia Acute dystonic reactions: torticollis, oculogyric crisis, ▲ muscle tone Tardive dyskinesia Hyperprolactinaemia amenorrhoea, galactorrhoea, sexual dysfunction, ▲ breast cancer	**Anticholinergic** Dry mouth urinary retention constipation confusion
Clozapine Hypersalivation constipation hypo/hypertension, weight gain, fever, nausea, nocturnal enuresis *Seizures* *Agranulocytosis*	**Phenothiazines** blood dyscrasias, retinal pigmentation, photosensitivity, cholestatic jaundice	**Cardiac** Prolonged QT interval arrhythmias 2x risk of sudden cardiac death **Neuroleptic malignant syndrome** hyperpyrexia, autonomic instability, confusion ▲ muscle tone, ▲ serum creatine phosphokinase **Antihistaminergic** sedation **Antiadrenergic** Postural hypotension (especially chlorpromazine) impotence

Figure 30.5 The main groups of antidepressants and their side effects

Antidepressant	Side effects	
Serotonin-noradrenergic reuptake inhibitors **Fluoxetine** **Citalopram** **Paroxetine** **Sertraline** **Fluvoxamine** **Serotonin-noradrenergic reuptake inhibitors** **Venlafaxine** **Duloxetine**	Headache Anorexia Nausea Indigestion Anxiety Sexual dysfunction ⚠ ↑ suicide ideation; not recommended < 18 years (except fluoxetine) ⚠ withdrawal syndrome	Selective Serotonin Reuptake Inhibitors mainly: ⚠ Gastrointestinal bleeding Hyponatraemia in older people Venlafaxine: Hypertension / hypotension Cardiotoxic in overdose
Noradrenergic and specific serotonergic antidepressant **Mirtazapine**	Dry mouth, drowsiness and weight gain	
Tricyclic antidepressants **Amitriptyline** **(dosulepin)** **Imipramine** **Lofepramine**	Anticholinergic Antiadrenergic ⚠ cardiac arrhythmias ⚠ seizures	
Monoamine oxidase Inhibitors **Phenelzine** **Tranylcypromine**	Anticholinergic Antiadrenergic Tyramine reaction	
Melatonergic agonist **Agomelatine**	Nausea, diarrhoea, constipation, abdominal pain Increased serum transaminases Headache, dizziness, drowsiness Anxiety, insomnia, fatigue Back pain Sweating	

Figure 30.6 Effects of lithium dosages

Below 0.4 mmol/L	0.4–1.0 mmol/L	Above 1.0 mmol/L
Ineffective	Therapeutic window	Toxic dose
	Side effects nausea fine tremor weight gain oedema polydipsia and polyuria exacerbation of psoriasis and acne hypothyroidism	**Signs of toxicity** vomiting diarrhoea coarse tremor slurred speech ataxia drowsiness and confusion convulsions and coma

then 6 months thereafter. As well as initially, serum lithium should be taken weekly and then every 12 weeks (Figure 30.6). Other mood stabilisers include sodium valproate and carbamazepine.

Antidementia drugs

Donepezil, rivastigmine, galantamine and memantine are used in the treatment of dementia.

Children

Psychiatric medication is frequently prescribed in the treatment of several psychiatric disorders in childhood such as nocturnal enuresis, attention-deficit hyperactivity disorder, autism, sleep disorders, tic disorders, conduct disorders, anxiety disorders, depression and psychosis. It is important to recognise that children differ from adults in their ability to absorb, metabolise and eliminate drugs.

Further reading

Royal College of Psychiatrists. Information on ECT.
    URL: http://www.rcpsych.ac.uk/expertadvice/
    treatmentswellbeing/ect.aspx
Mind. Drugs – an alphabetical list. URL: http://www.mind.org.uk/
    mental_health_a-z/8056_drugs_an_alphabetical_list
Pandya, S. (2009) Antipsychotics: uses, actions and prescribing
    rationale. *Nurse Prescribing* 7(1): 23–7.

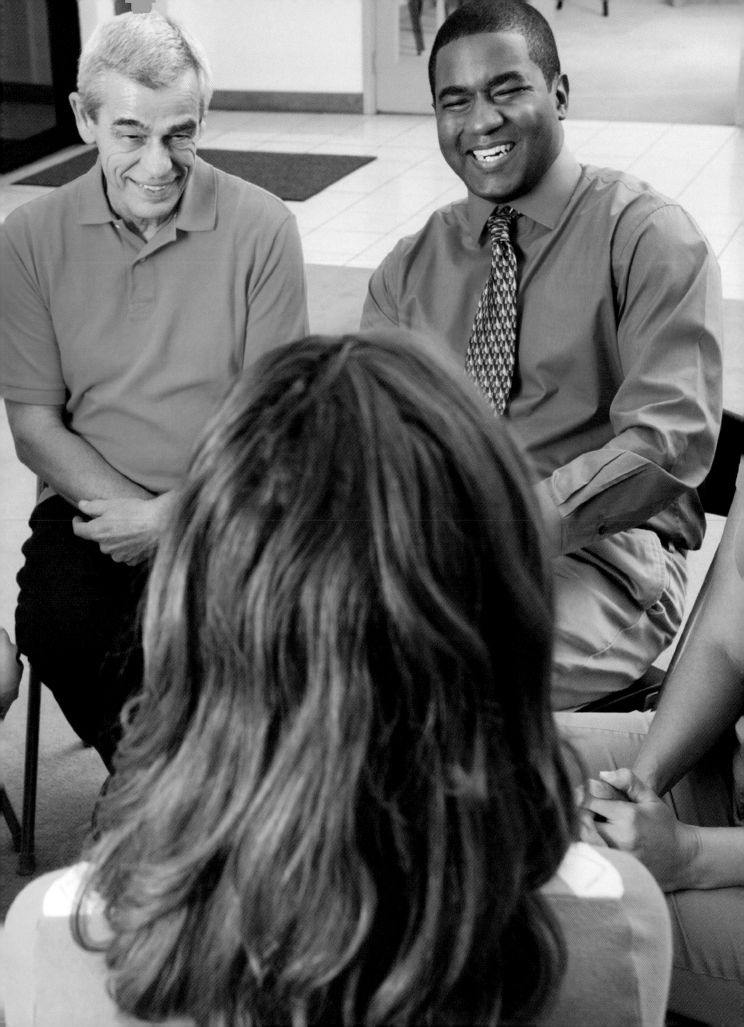

Leadership skills

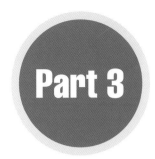

Part 3

Chapters

31 **Organising care** 72
32 **Leadership** 74
33 **Managing people** 76
34 **Time management** 78
35 **Decision-making** 80
36 **Utilising research** 82
37 **Reflection** 84
38 **Lifelong learning** 86

Don't forget to visit the companion website for this book www.ataglanceseries.com/nursing/mentalhealth to do some practice MCQs and case studies on these topics.

31 Organising care

Figure 31.1 The practice tree: Organising care

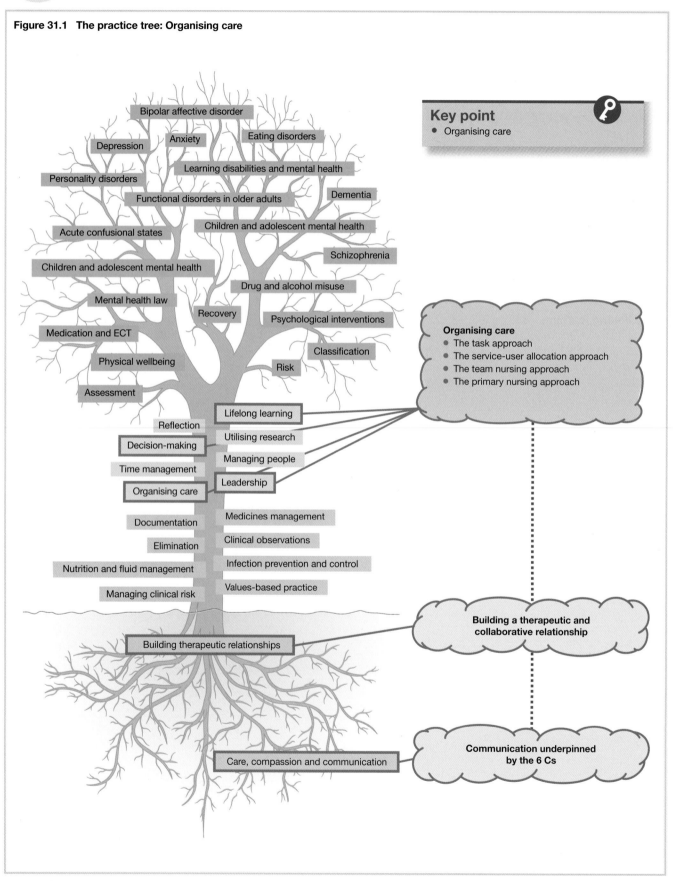

Key point
- Organising care

Bipolar affective disorder

Anxiety

Depression

Eating disorders

Learning disabilities and mental health

Personality disorders

Functional disorders in older adults

Dementia

Acute confusional states

Children and adolescent mental health

Children and adolescent mental health

Schizophrenia

Mental health law

Drug and alcohol misuse

Recovery

Medication and ECT

Psychological interventions

Physical wellbeing

Classification

Risk

Assessment

Organising care
- The task approach
- The service-user allocation approach
- The team nursing approach
- The primary nursing approach

Lifelong learning

Reflection

Utilising research

Decision-making

Managing people

Time management

Leadership

Organising care

Documentation

Medicines management

Elimination

Clinical observations

Nutrition and fluid management

Infection prevention and control

Managing clinical risk

Values-based practice

Building therapeutic relationships

Building a therapeutic and collaborative relationship

Care, compassion and communication

Communication underpinned by the 6 Cs

Mental Health Nursing at a Glance, First Edition. Grahame Smith. © 2015 John Wiley & Sons, Ltd. Published 2015 by John Wiley & Sons, Ltd.
Companion website: www.ataglanceseries.com/nursing/mentalhealth

Introduction

Mental health nurses are professionally accountable for their own practice, but they rarely work in isolation. Most mental health nurses will work as part of a multiprofessional team but they may also work as part of a nursing team. Within these different teams care delivery decisions will be made and acted upon. During this process the mental health nurse needs to be both an effective team leader and an effective team member. They also need to ensure that the service user is at the centre of the decision-making process where their rights are fully respected.

Competencies

Mental health nurses are required to:
• Work as an autonomous and confident member of the multiprofessional team who promotes the continuity of care.
• Safely lead, coordinate and manage care that is responsive to the needs of individuals living with mental health problems.
• Deliver personalised care that is based on mutual understanding and respect for the individual's situation.
• Maintain a safe environment and safeguard individuals living with mental health problems from vulnerable and potentially harmful situations.

The context

Health and social care structures appear to be constantly changing both at a national and at a local level. Organisational structures that are constantly changing can at an operational level impact upon the way care is delivered. The role of the mental health nurse is to negotiate this constant change while delivering the best care available. An added challenge for the mental health nurse is the fluidity of organisational structures within the mental health field especially where there is a greater focus on community working and multidisciplinary case management. The structure of an organisation is dependent on the organisation's aims; for example, mental health NHS trusts aim to provide health and social care for individuals with mental health problems. This provision is delivered through a number of services which include:
• forensic;
• drugs and alcohol;
• acute in-patient;
• liaison psychiatry;
• community mental health;
• crisis intervention;
• assertive outreach;
• early intervention;
• outreach;
• rehabilitation.

Organising care delivery

Different models are used to organise mental health nursing care. Whatever model is used it should always aim to provide a good quality of care. Within an in-patient environment the delivery of

this care is influenced by the multidisciplinary decision-making process; this may be via multidisciplinary team meetings or ward rounds. At an operational level nurses deliver the majority of this care, and organise care delivery (Figure 31.1) through a number of different approaches; however, these approaches are not mutually exclusive:
• The task approach – the focus will be on delivering tasks such as administering medication or undertaking observations.
• The service-user allocation approach – a nurse will be assigned to care for a specific number of service users.
• The team nursing approach – a team of qualified and unqualified nurses will care for a specific group of service users.
• The primary nursing approach – a service user throughout their stay in hospital will be cared for by a named qualified nurse who will be responsible and accountable for the coordination of their care.

A case management approach to care delivery is typically used within the community mental health team settings. It is a multidisciplinary team approach where a number of professional groups are involved in both the decision-making process and the delivery of care, though in terms of overall responsibility one member of the team is allocated to be the case manager.

Person-centred care

Whatever the model used, nursing care delivery should aim to be person-centred, focusing on the service user's needs, strengths and preferences. It should also take into account that a service user may lack capacity and in this case the mental health nurse should follow the relevant legal framework/guidance.

Best practice

Mental health nurses while working in partnership with service users who have complex needs are required to deliver high-quality care. During this process they also have to be able to successfully influence external agencies to ensure that a holistic and integrated package of care is effectively implemented. As an added dimension they will at the same time have to make sense of a health and social care environment where structures are constantly changing. Using a model of care delivery will provide a sense of consistency when dealing with all this change, though it is important that the nurse is skilful enough to adapt to different ways of working. On this basis the nurse will have to complement their baseline skills by engaging in a journey of lifelong learning where they clearly identify and address their identified learning needs.

Further reading

Department of Health (2010) Front Line Care: the future of nursing and midwifery in England. Report of the Prime Minister's Commission on the Future of Nursing and Midwifery in England 2010. London: Department of Health.

Department of Health (2012) Vision and Strategy: An Approach to the Nursing and Midwifery Contribution of 'No Health Without Mental Health'. London: Department of Health.

McKenzie, C. & Manley, K. (2011) Leadership and responsive care: Principle of Nursing Practice H. *Nursing Standard* 25(35): 35–7.

32 Leadership

Figure 32.1 The practice tree: Leadership

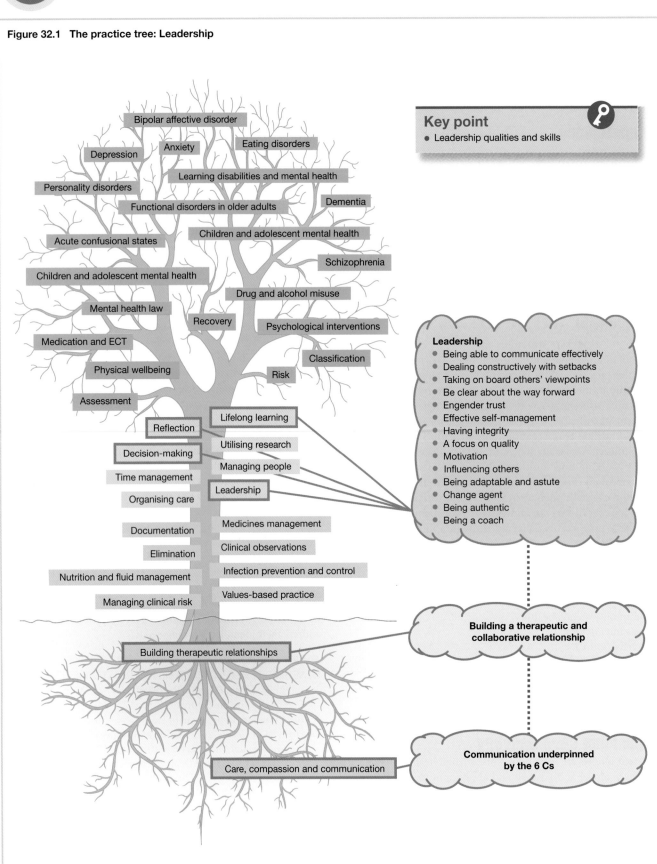

Key point
- Leadership qualities and skills

Leadership
- Being able to communicate effectively
- Dealing constructively with setbacks
- Taking on board others' viewpoints
- Be clear about the way forward
- Engender trust
- Effective self-management
- Having integrity
- A focus on quality
- Motivation
- Influencing others
- Being adaptable and astute
- Change agent
- Being authentic
- Being a coach

Building a therapeutic and collaborative relationship

Communication underpinned by the 6 Cs

Mental Health Nursing at a Glance, First Edition. Grahame Smith. © 2015 John Wiley & Sons, Ltd. Published 2015 by John Wiley & Sons, Ltd.
Companion website: www.ataglanceseries.com/nursing/mentalhealth

Introduction

Management and leadership are terms that are generally used synonymously; management usually describes the administrative aspect whereas leadership is used in a much broader way. It is easy to think that leadership is about being in a specific leadership role or formal role when in reality it is usually about assuming an informal leadership role when care delivery dictates. For example, the nurse may take a lead role within a multidisciplinary team meeting advocating a specific treatment on behalf of a service user. At a professional level leadership is a developmental journey that should focus on the nurse being able to positively contribute to the delivery of high-quality care.

Competencies

Mental health nurses are required to:
• Be able to manage themselves and others to ensure the quality of care and the safety of the service user are maintained or enhanced.
• Be self-aware and professionally accountable using clinical governance processes to maintain and improve practice standards.
• Work effectively across professional and agency boundaries to create and maximise opportunities to help improve the care delivery.
• Actively participate in further developing their management and leadership skills through structured reflection.

The context

Effective leadership within health and social care is viewed as a key component in the drive to improve care quality. To do this mental health nurses must be able to work in partnership with individuals living with mental health problems, other professionals and external agencies. During this process they must also be able to lead effectively (see Figure 32.1) through the utilisation of leadership skills, behaviours and values, which include:
• being able to communicate effectively;
• dealing constructively with setbacks;
• taking on board others' viewpoints;
• being clear about the way forward;
• engendering trust.

Depending on the situation the mental health nurse may use different leadership styles. For example, in an emergency situation the nurse's actions might be more directive (autocratic style) rather than seeking everyone's view (democratic style) or just allowing everyone to do their own thing (laissez-faire style).

Models of leadership

There are a number of theories and models of leadership, which include:
• Traits-based leadership – leaders are born not made, and they are born with the personality traits to be leaders.

• Leadership as a behavioural style – leadership behaviours should be applied depending on the situation; as a behavioural skill some situations might require the leader to demonstrate decisiveness, other situations may not.
• Situational-contingency approaches to leadership – a leader is required to adapt their leadership style to suit the situation or circumstances: at times they may be required to be an authoritarian team leader and at other times they may seek the advice of the team.
• Transformational approaches – a leader focuses on enhancing the performance of individuals they lead through a number of different approaches such as motivating individuals, providing a vision or direction, and through being a role model.

Improving practice

Clinical leadership should focus on continually improving the quality of care delivered to mental health service users. This is irrespective of whether a mental health nurse's leadership role is informal or formal. To establish a strong foundation for being an effective clinical leader it is useful if the mental health nurse develops their practice to a level where they can skilfully cope with a range of clinical situations. Building on this foundation through lifelong learning the mental health nurse as a leader (Figure 32.1) should consider cultivating the following qualities:
• effective self-management;
• having integrity;
• a focus on quality;
• motivation;
• influencing others;
• being adaptable and astute;
• change agent;
• being authentic;
• being a coach.

The roles of mental health nurse and clinical leader embody similar skills, values and qualities. To ensure that these are cultivated and directed in the right direction the mental health nurse as a practitioner and as a leader should actively engage in:
• lifelong learning;
• expert skill development;
• critical reflection.

Further reading

Foundation of Nursing Leadership. URL: http://www.nursingleadership.org.uk/

Goleman, D. (1998) What makes a leader? In: Henry, J. (ed.) (2006) *Creative Management Development*, 3rd edn. London: Sage Publications.

NHS Leadership Academy. Leadership Framework. URL: http://www.leadershipacademy.nhs.uk/discover/leadership-framework/

Managing people

Figure 33.1 The practice tree: Managing people

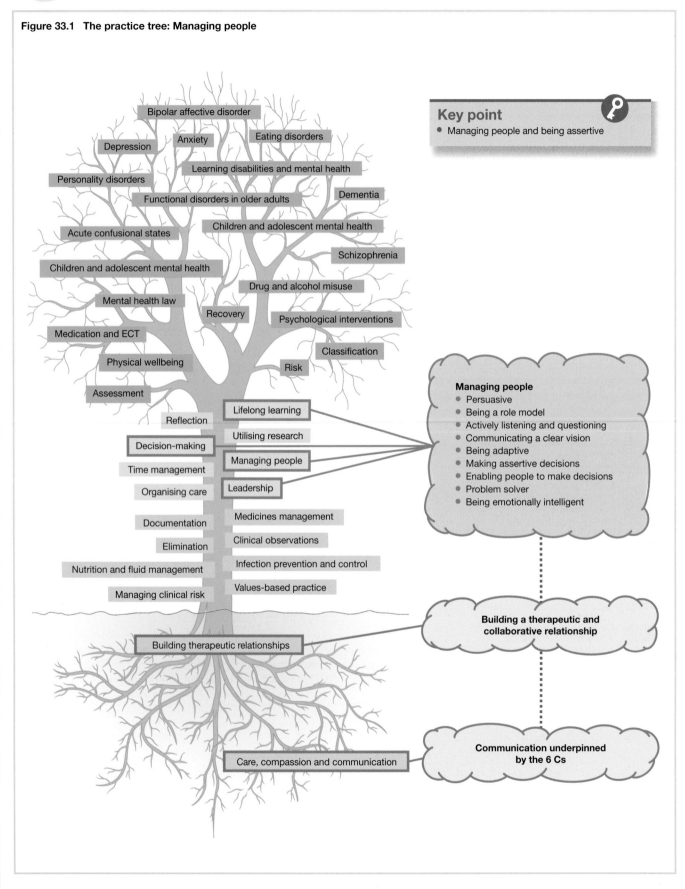

Key point
- Managing people and being assertive

Managing people
- Persuasive
- Being a role model
- Actively listening and questioning
- Communicating a clear vision
- Being adaptive
- Making assertive decisions
- Enabling people to make decisions
- Problem solver
- Being emotionally intelligent

Building a therapeutic and collaborative relationship

Communication underpinned by the 6 Cs

Tree labels:
Bipolar affective disorder
Depression · Anxiety · Eating disorders
Personality disorders · Learning disabilities and mental health
Functional disorders in older adults · Dementia
Acute confusional states · Children and adolescent mental health
Children and adolescent mental health · Schizophrenia
Mental health law · Drug and alcohol misuse
Recovery · Psychological interventions
Medication and ECT · Classification
Physical wellbeing · Risk
Assessment
Reflection · Lifelong learning
Decision-making · Utilising research
Time management · Managing people
Organising care · Leadership
Documentation · Medicines management
Elimination · Clinical observations
Nutrition and fluid management · Infection prevention and control
Managing clinical risk · Values-based practice
Building therapeutic relationships
Care, compassion and communication

Mental Health Nursing at a Glance, First Edition. Grahame Smith. © 2015 John Wiley & Sons, Ltd. Published 2015 by John Wiley & Sons, Ltd.
Companion website: www.ataglanceseries.com/nursing/mentalhealth

Introduction

Part of the role of the mental health nurse is to manage others, whether in a formal or informal capacity. Before the nurse starts to manage others they first have to be able to manage themselves; key to this is self-awareness. By being self-aware the nurse is not only aware of their thoughts and feelings, they should in time be able to understand how they affect others. Furthermore, as they become skilled in understanding self and others then dynamically the next stage is to use the self to influence and facilitate positive change. During this process the nurse will also become assertive, in which they are neither aggressive – imposing their will on others – nor submissive – allowing others to impose their will on them.

Competencies

Mental health nurses are required to:
- Manage themselves and others effectively.
- Work collaboratively with mental health service users, carers, other professionals and agencies to enhance care delivery.
- Actively engage in lifelong learning both as a practitioner and as a leader to enhance care.
- Assertively challenge the practice of self and others.
- Act as an effective role model and as an effective clinical supervisor during the care delivery process.

The context

During recent times the formal role of managing nursing teams has become more complex. Not only are there many different nursing management roles but it is not always clear from a title what they do or do not manage. Also management roles within health and social care can change almost overnight. However, there are some common management functions, which may include:
- managing the performance of a team and individuals;
- delegation;
- resolving conflict;
- managing change;
- decision-making.

At an informal level where a nurse is part of a team but is leading on issue such as advocating on behalf of a service user, the nurse needs to be an effective influencer (see Figure 33.1). This is especially the case where they need to change the attitudes of others to gain an agreed position or way forward. Influencing skills include:
- active listening and questioning;
- persuasion;
- being assertive.

People management skills

Managing people can be stressful but it can also be rewarding. The key to being effective in this role is preparation. This can take the form of a formal course and/or being mentored in the process of developing effective managing people skills. The types of skills (Figure 33.1) the mental nurse would look to develop include:
- being a role model;
- actively listening to people;
- communicating a clear vision of the way forward;
- being adaptive – use different skills for different situations;
- making assertive decisions;
- enabling people to make decisions;
- taking a systematic approach to problem solving;
- being emotionally intelligent.

Coaching and mentoring

Mental health nurses during their day-to-day role will support and mentor students; this is a process where the nurse supports the student in the course of achieving a number of set goals. To do this the nurse will facilitate the student's learning through a systematic process where they will:
- role model a skill;
- give the student an opportunity to safely practise the skill;
- support the student to carry out the skill in live practice;
- provide structured feedback;
- engage the student in critical thinking.

Coaching can be a similar process though there is less focus on the teaching aspect and more focus on improving performance through an action-focused dialogue. The coaching relationship gives the coachee the opportunity to have protected space to focus on their development, which is similar in some aspects to the clinical supervision process/relationship. The mental health nurse as a coachee may utilise this approach to develop their own people management skills or they may coach others to develop their skills. Coaching can also be used as way of ensuring that individuals (coachees) are accountable for their development through the setting of agreed actions and outcomes, it can also be used to support individuals through change.

Managing change

Change can have an emotional impact, which needs to be managed by a leader who is sensitive to this emotional context. A way of doing this is by seeing the role of managing people through change as more about managing relationships and building support than just driving through change. In this situation the mental health nurse needs to engage in a discussion with the individuals they manage in a way that is about negotiation and agreement, but is also:
- collaborative;
- productive;
- positive.

Further reading

Bowers, B. (2011) Managing change by empowering staff. *Nursing Times* **107**(32/33): 19–21.
Gopee, N. (2011) *Mentoring and Supervision in Healthcare*, 2nd edn. London, Sage.
Kline, R. (2013) Safe to delegate? *Nursing Standard* **27**(26): 19.

34 Time management

Figure 34.1   The practice tree: Time management

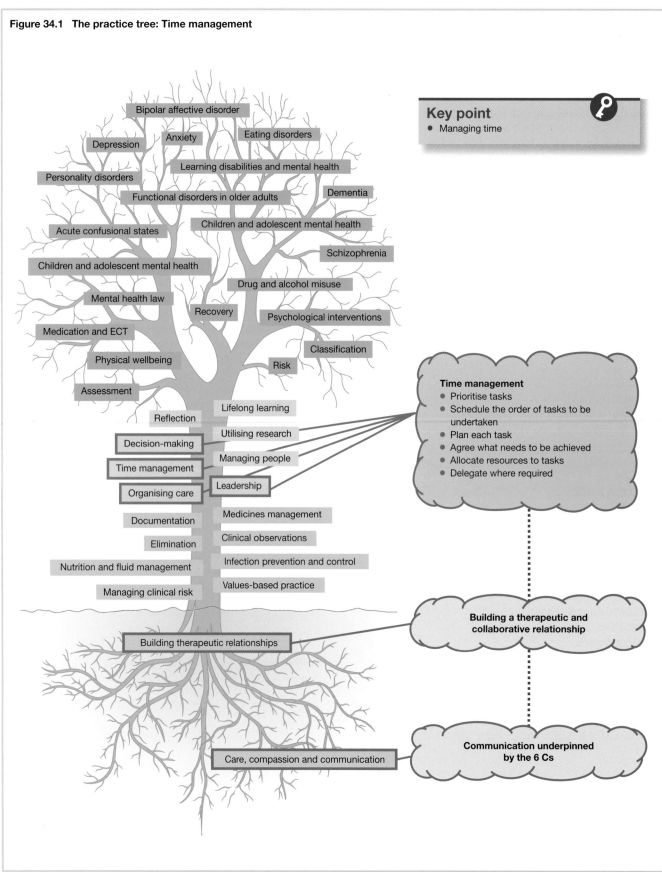

Key point
- Managing time

Time management
- Prioritise tasks
- Schedule the order of tasks to be undertaken
- Plan each task
- Agree what needs to be achieved
- Allocate resources to tasks
- Delegate where required

Building a therapeutic and collaborative relationship

Communication underpinned by the 6 Cs

Tree labels:
Bipolar affective disorder · Anxiety · Eating disorders · Depression · Learning disabilities and mental health · Personality disorders · Functional disorders in older adults · Dementia · Acute confusional states · Children and adolescent mental health · Schizophrenia · Children and adolescent mental health · Drug and alcohol misuse · Mental health law · Recovery · Psychological interventions · Medication and ECT · Classification · Physical wellbeing · Risk · Assessment · Lifelong learning · Reflection · Utilising research · Decision-making · Managing people · Time management · Leadership · Organising care · Medicines management · Documentation · Clinical observations · Elimination · Infection prevention and control · Nutrition and fluid management · Values-based practice · Managing clinical risk · Building therapeutic relationships · Care, compassion and communication

Mental Health Nursing at a Glance, First Edition. Grahame Smith. © 2015 John Wiley & Sons, Ltd. Published 2015 by John Wiley & Sons, Ltd.
Companion website: www.ataglanceseries.com/nursing/mentalhealth

Introduction

Mental health nurses in the process of delivering have to manage their time effectively. Time management is a complex process; it is not just about how the mental health nurse manages their time as a series of tasks; it is also about how they emotionally manage time pressure. A nurse who is an expert in a certain intervention may take less time than someone who is new to this intervention. This in itself is not problematic; the problem arises when the team expectation is that everyone can complete this intervention in the same amount of time. If a nurse cannot they can feel rushed or they rush to complete the intervention and consequently feel stressed. Another issue is that the delivery of mental health nursing care can be routine focused, with tasks planned in advance; but that routine has to be flexible as unexpected issues can arise that have to be dealt with, there and then.

Competencies

Mental health nurses are required to:
- Identify priorities and manage time and resources effectively to ensure the quality of care is maintained or enhanced.
- Prioritise the needs of groups and individuals in order to provide care effectively and efficiently.
- Negotiate with others in relation to balancing competing and conflicting priorities.
- Prioritise their own workload and manage competing and conflicting priorities.

The context

Care delivery has become increasingly complex with the mental nurse needing to manage many competing priorities. Managing time focuses on controlling the amount of time and effort spent on a specific task or intervention (Figure 34.1); this includes:
- prioritising tasks;
- scheduling the order of task to be undertaken;
- planning each task ;
- agreeing what needs to be achieved;
- allocating resources to the task;
- delegating where required.

Being systematic can be extremely helpful in managing time, but as health and social care provision can rapidly change it is important that this approach is flexible. Prioritisation should be the mediating factor in this flexible approach; for example, writing a care plan may well be a priority until an emergency situation arises on the ward. On this basis the mental health nurse should:
- be aware of what are priorities and what are not;
- set priorities being aware that they can change;
- deliver care based on those priorities.

Delegation

Where there is a team delivering care then tasks need to be allocated. The person undertaking the task should be the "best person for the job". It would be nice if the team allocated their own tasks but usually it falls to the team leader. The appropriate and safe use of delegation can create a sense of time and space: "one person does not feel they are doing everything". When delegating, the following have to be considered:
- Does the person have the right skills and knowledge?
- Are they legally allowed to undertake the task?
- What does the organisation's policy say?
- Who is accountable and responsible?
- Does the person know exactly what they need to do?
- Is delegating the task the best option?

Stress management

One benefit of being a good time manager is that it helps the mental health nurse cope with stress in a way that is healthy. Stress in itself is not a bad thing; it is usually transient, and at times we all feel a bit stressed. It becomes problematic when the mental or emotional pressure adversely impacts upon an individual's ability to function healthily; in other words an individual may feel unable to cope. People have different stress levels and different ways of coping; therefore it is important for the mental health nurse to recognise when they are stressed and whether it is having a negative impact upon their ability to cope. Prolonged stress manifests in different ways:
- sleep problems;
- loss of appetite;
- difficulty in concentrating;
- constantly feeling anxious;
- feeing irritable and/or angry;
- having repeating thoughts;
- worrying;
- avoiding certain situations and/or people;
- an increased use of alcohol;
- headaches;
- muscle tension.

Prolonged stress can lead to the individual experiencing emotional exhaustion, and in some cases leading to a number of mental disorders. To manage stress consider the following activities:
- engage in physical activity;
- engage in something that makes you laugh;
- learn relaxation and/or deep breathing techniques;
- take control of the situation;
- seek support and talk;
- problem solve;
- eat healthily;
- drink plenty of water;
- be mindful.

Further reading

Redfern Jones, J. (2012) Time is on your side. *Nursing Standard* **26**(38): 70–1.

Royal College of Nursing (2005) *Managing your Stress: A Guide for Nurses*. London: RCN.

Waterworth, S. (2003) Time management strategies in nursing practice. *Journal of Advanced Nursing* **43**(5): 432–40.

35 Decision-making

Figure 35.1 The practice tree: Decision-making

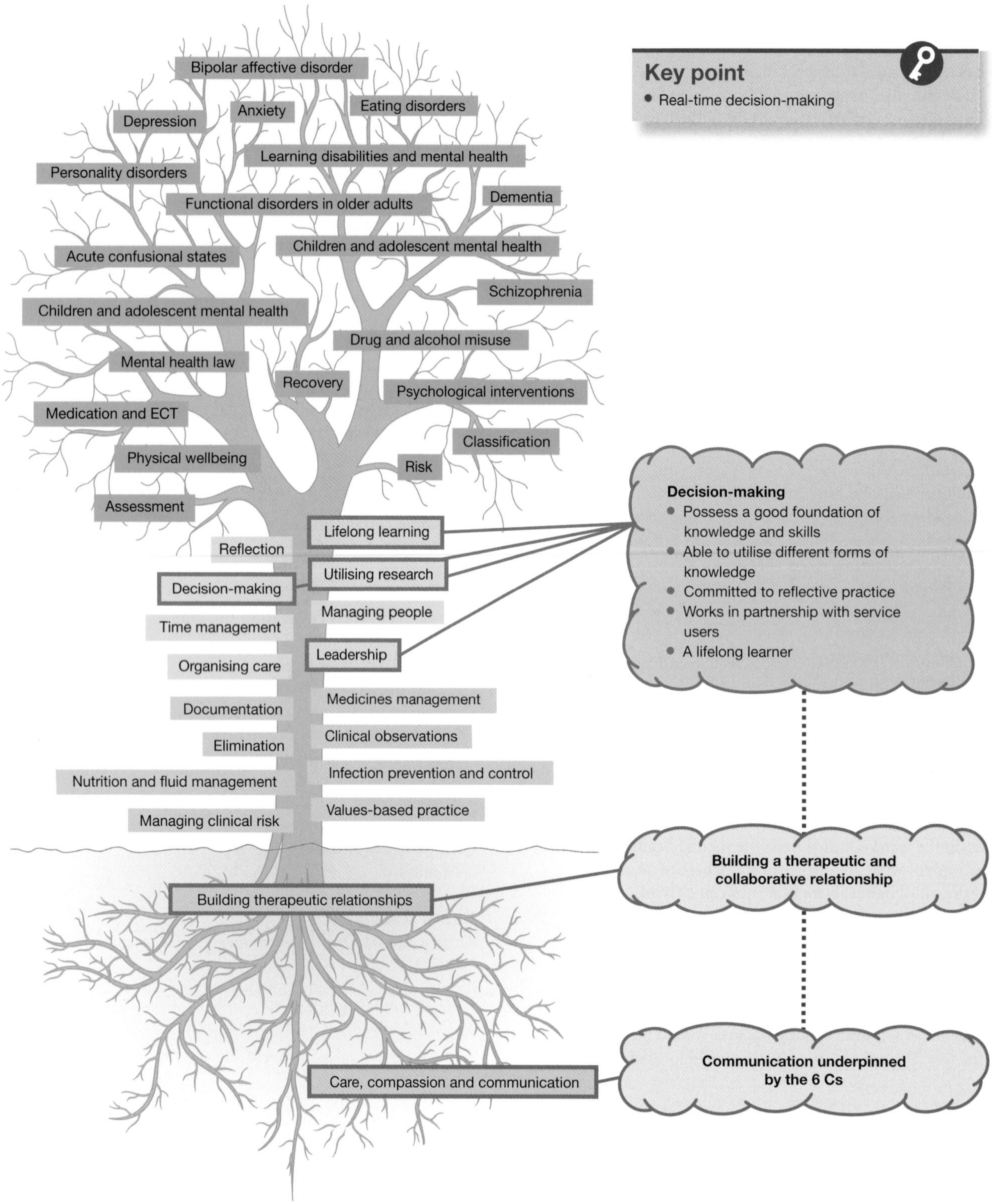

Bipolar affective disorder

Anxiety

Eating disorders

Depression

Personality disorders

Learning disabilities and mental health

Functional disorders in older adults

Dementia

Acute confusional states

Children and adolescent mental health

Children and adolescent mental health

Schizophrenia

Mental health law

Drug and alcohol misuse

Recovery

Psychological interventions

Medication and ECT

Classification

Physical wellbeing

Risk

Assessment

Lifelong learning

Reflection

Utilising research

Decision-making

Managing people

Time management

Leadership

Organising care

Documentation

Medicines management

Elimination

Clinical observations

Nutrition and fluid management

Infection prevention and control

Managing clinical risk

Values-based practice

Building therapeutic relationships

Care, compassion and communication

Key point
- Real-time decision-making

Decision-making
- Possess a good foundation of knowledge and skills
- Able to utilise different forms of knowledge
- Committed to reflective practice
- Works in partnership with service users
- A lifelong learner

Building a therapeutic and collaborative relationship

Communication underpinned by the 6 Cs

Introduction

Mental health nurses are organisationally and professionally accountable for the practice decisions they make. These decisions are made on a day-to-day basis, some being more complex than others. Irrespective of their complexity the nurse needs to be able to justify these decisions. On this basis clinical decisions should be evidence-based, with nurse being able to explain which evidence they use and why. Being transparent in this way should not just be a means to an end, such as defending a decision, it should also be a process where making clinical decisions involves other professionals and more importantly individuals living with mental health problems.

Competencies

Mental health nurses are required to:
• Ensure that clinical decision-making is person-centred and evidence-based and the outcomes of this process are evaluated.
• Make decisions in partnership with others involved in the care process to ensure high-quality care.
• Signpost to others when the complexity of clinical decisions requires specialist knowledge and expertise.
• Recognise and address the ethical context of clinical decision-making in a way that focuses on agreed and acceptable solutions.

The context

When delivering care mental health nurses have to be effective decision makers. This need for effective clinical decision-making is driven by a quality process where there is an expectation that care delivery is of a high standard and nurses are publically accountable for the clinical decisions they make. To make a clinical decision the mental health nurse needs to:
• identify the issue/s;
• analyse the evidence;
• consider the options;
• plan a way forward;
• implement the decision;
• evaluate the outcome.
Making a decision in this way can appear logical and unemotional, but it is important to note that decision-making in clinical practice will most of the time have an emotional context. That is why the evaluation of the decision is so vital and should be linked into the nurse's reflective practices. Certainly for mental health nurses as there is a values-based context to practice there is a need also to be ethically sensitive especially when dealing with the sensitive issue of restricting a service user's freedoms.

Analysing the evidence

Analysing and using the best evidence is a key part of the clinical decision-making process. The focus of this approach is to provide the best care available. Using the best evidence ensures that established care delivery is also underpinned by research-based evidence; the evidence used in this approach is usually scientific evidence. Utilising evidence-based knowledge in clinical decision-making requires the mental health nurse to be able to:
• succinctly identify the clinical issue ;
• understand the issue as a clinical question ;
• search the literature;
• critique different forms of evidence;
• deliver the chosen intervention;
• evaluate the delivery of the intervention.
Further to choosing a specific intervention the mental health nurse will also have to consider whether this intervention can be situated within the therapeutic relationship in a way that reflects the specific needs of the mental health service user.

Challenges

Decisions are not made in isolation; there are a number of influencing factors the mental health nurse has to take into consideration, which include:
• Is there enough information available to make an effective decision?
• What are the timescales?
• What are you trying to achieve?
• Are the required skills and resources available to implement the chosen intervention?
• What are the risks of either taking action or not taking action?

Real-time decisions

Systematic approaches to decision-making can be useful though it has to be accepted that a number of clinical decisions have to be made in real time (Figure 35.1). For example, a mental health service user may be actively seeking to harm themselves; in this situation the mental health nurse will need to act quickly and "keep the service user safe". Acting quickly is not an excuse for not doing the right thing, and on this basis the mental health nurse will need to ensure that they are properly prepared to be able to effectively deal with this type of situation. Being properly prepared stems from:
• having a good foundation of knowledge and skills;
• being able to utilise different forms of knowledge such as scientific, naturalistic, personal and ethical knowledge;
• having the commitment to engage in reflective practice that is structured and protected;
• working in true partnership with mental health service users;
• being a lifelong learner.

Further reading

Banning, M. (2008) A review of clinical decision making: models and current research. *Journal of Clinical Nursing* **17**: 187–95.

Crook, J.A. (2001) How do expert nurses make on-the-spot clinical decisions? A review of the literature. *Journal of Psychiatric and Mental Health Nursing* **8**: 1–5.

Welsh, I. & Lyons, C.M. (2001) Evidence-based care and the case for intuition and tacit knowledge in clinical assessment and decision making in mental health nursing practice: an empirical contribution to the debate. *Journal of Psychiatric and Mental Health Nursing* **8**: 299–305.

36 Utilising research

Figure 36.1   The practice tree: Utilising research

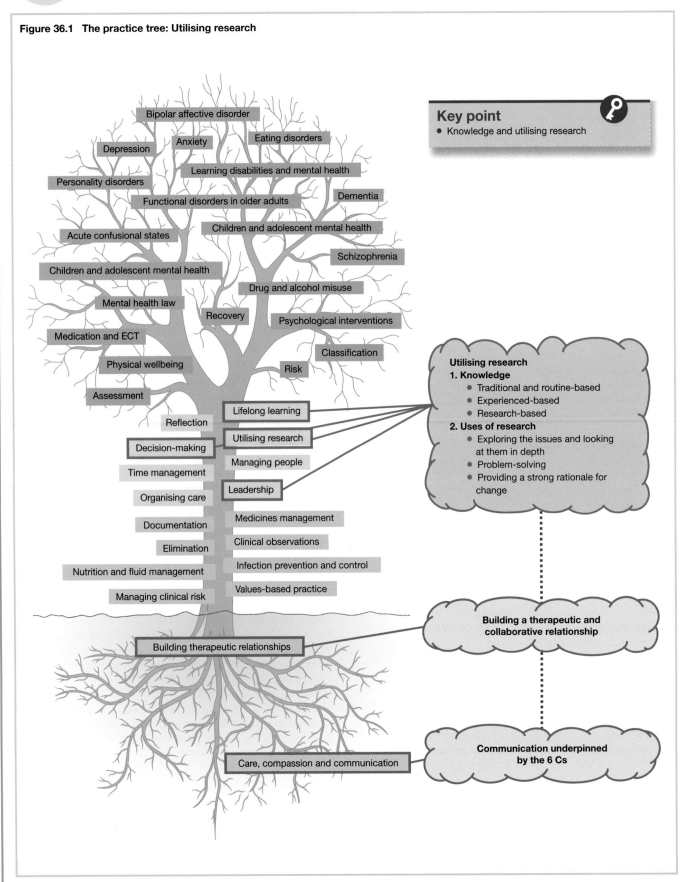

Key point
- Knowledge and utilising research

Utilising research
1. Knowledge
- Traditional and routine-based
- Experienced-based
- Research-based

2. Uses of research
- Exploring the issues and looking at them in depth
- Problem-solving
- Providing a strong rationale for change

Building a therapeutic and collaborative relationship

Communication underpinned by the 6 Cs

Tree labels:
Bipolar affective disorder
Depression
Anxiety
Eating disorders
Personality disorders
Learning disabilities and mental health
Functional disorders in older adults
Dementia
Acute confusional states
Children and adolescent mental health
Children and adolescent mental health
Schizophrenia
Drug and alcohol misuse
Mental health law
Recovery
Psychological interventions
Medication and ECT
Classification
Physical wellbeing
Risk
Assessment
Lifelong learning
Reflection
Utilising research
Decision-making
Managing people
Time management
Leadership
Organising care
Documentation
Medicines management
Elimination
Clinical observations
Nutrition and fluid management
Infection prevention and control
Managing clinical risk
Values-based practice
Building therapeutic relationships
Care, compassion and communication

Mental Health Nursing at a Glance, First Edition. Grahame Smith. © 2015 John Wiley & Sons, Ltd. Published 2015 by John Wiley & Sons, Ltd.
Companion website: www.ataglanceseries.com/nursing/mentalhealth

Introduction

Utilising good quality research evidence will assist the mental health nurse in providing a continuing high standard of care with improved care outcomes. To utilise such evidence effectively and appropriately the nurse will need to be competent in the use of research-based evidence. Part of being competent relates to knowing what evidence is useful and what evidence is not so useful and also being able to justify the decision taken. It is worth noting that there are different forms of knowledge though in terms of clinical guidelines scientific evidence is the key form of knowledge used in mental health nursing practice.

Competencies

Mental health nurses are required to:
• Deliver care that is responsive to the needs of individuals living with mental health problems and is appropriately based on research evidence.
• Ensure their practice is informed by the best available evidence and complies with local and national guidelines.
• Recognise the value of evidence in practice and be able to understand and appraise research, apply relevant theory and research findings to practice, and identify areas for further investigation.
• Use research-based evidence to assist in improving mental health service users' care experiences and care outcomes and also to shape future care provision.

The context

Nursing practice (Figure 36.1) utilises different types of knowledge:
• traditional and routine-based;
• experienced-based;
• research-based.
The nurse will not exclusively use one source of knowledge. As an example, research may suggest that the nurse should change their practice in a certain way; experience may further modify this change, which then becomes the norm or traditional practice. Research is a systematic way of gaining knowledge where what is already known is either added to, rejected or confirmed. It can assist the nurse (see Figure 36.1) in the process of:
• exploring the issues and looking at them in depth;
• problem-solving;
• providing a strong rationale for change.
Generally research can be quantitative, focusing on measuring and cause and effect; or qualitative, which is more concerned with value-laden or subjective issues.

Scientific evidence

Scientific or quantitative evidence and approaches take different forms though the dominant form in mental health nursing practice is the evidence-based form, or what is called evidence-based practice (EBP). This relates to the clinical decision-making process being based on the careful use of current and best evidence.

This evidence can range from testimony from a clinical expert to evidence that is collected through randomised controlled trials (RCTs). The ideal type is evidence that is collected through the RCT process. It is important to note that this type of evidence is continually being updated, and on this basis the nurse needs to ensure that they too are regularly updated about any changes. This should include checking any relevant clinical guidelines that are shaped by EBP as the guidelines change as the evidence changes. EBP has number of steps, starting with asking a clinical question such as "what is the best nursing intervention for this condition?" The nurse will then move on to:
• identifying the relevant literature that helps address the question;
• critically assessing the evidence – is it reliable and/or valid?
• applying the chosen evidence;
• evaluating the application of the evidence.

Naturalistic evidence

Qualitative or naturalistic research is interested in researching experiences and meanings, such as why individuals act in the way they do. The different types of naturalistic research approaches include:
• phenomenology;
• grounded theory;
• ethnography;
• narrative studies;
• case studies.
In terms of these approaches the most commonly used methods of collecting information are:
• interviews;
• narratives;
• case studies;
• focus groups.

Practice evidence

EBP may be a dominant approach though it is important to recognise that scientific knowledge only provides one perspective, which can be a limited way of understanding a service user's mental distress. A better understanding can be engendered through multiple meanings, which may include working with both EBP information and also the service user's narrative. Working in this manner with both scientific and naturalistic knowledge assists the nurse in having a more holistic understanding of a mental health service user's needs.

Further reading

Callaghan, P. & Crawford, P. (2009) Evidence-based mental health nursing practice. In: Callaghan, P., Playle, J. & Cooper, L. (eds) *Mental Health Nursing Skills*. Oxford: Oxford University Press, pp. 33–43.

Franks, V. (2004) Evidence-based uncertainty in mental health nursing. *Journal of Psychiatric and Mental Health Nursing* **11**: 99–105.

Parahoo, K. (2006) *Nursing Research: Principles, Process and Issues*, 2nd edn. Basingstoke: Palgrave Macmillan.

37 Reflection

Figure 37.1 The practice tree: Reflection

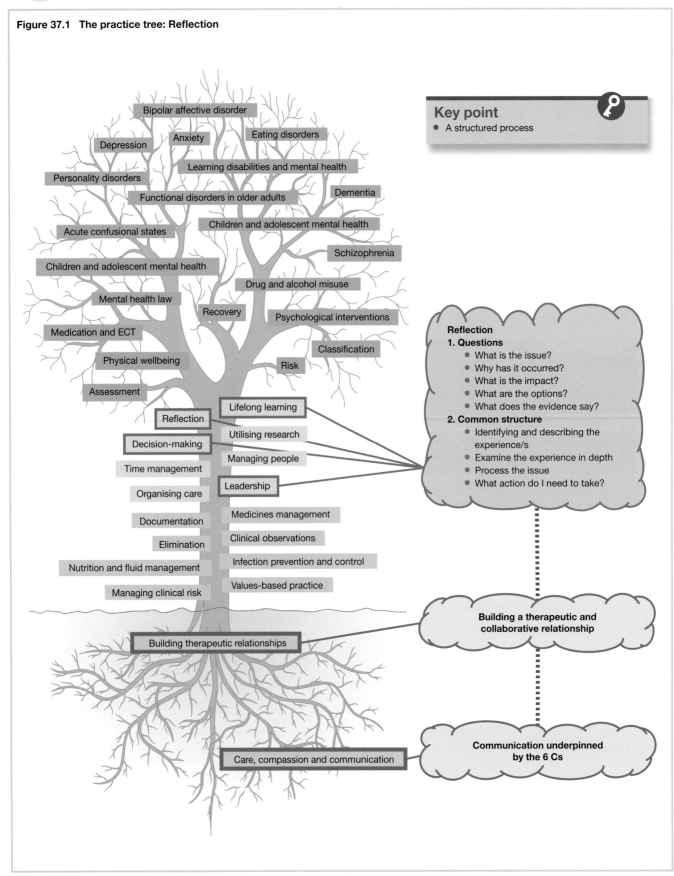

Introduction

Mental health nurses are professionally required to engage in the process of reflection, the most common form being reflection on action, which relates to thinking and feeling about practice experiences in a way that promotes learning. For this process to be effective the nurse needs to be committed to a better understanding of their own values and how these relate to the values of the nursing profession. They also need to be committed to constantly improving their practice. A common method of systematically reflecting on practice is through clinical supervision, which is a formal activity where a clinical supervisor facilitates the nurse to reflect upon their practice and identify strategies that focus on improving their practice.

Competencies

Mental health nurses are required to:
• Actively participate in clinical supervision and reflection.
• Engage in reflection and supervision to ensure they learn from their practice experiences in a way that enhances the quality of care they provide.
• Participate in the reflective process as a mechanism to better understand their personal values, beliefs and emotions and how they can impact upon their practice.
• Actively promote clinical supervision as clinical leader and as clinical role model.

The context

The professional expectation is that the mental health nurse at the point of registration is a critically reflective practitioner who learns from practice in a way that improves the quality of the care they deliver. Being critically reflective implies that the nurse is able to identify critical incidents that arise from their practice experiences. This essentially is a questioning process (see Figure 37.1) where the nurse would consider:
• What is the issue, is it problematic and why?
• Why has it occurred?
• How does this issue impact upon the service user?
• What are the options or alternatives?
• Have you looked at the evidence?
     The skills of critical reflection arise from engaging in reflection in two interconnected forms:
• Reflection on action – reflecting after an experience and then taking action to improve practice.
• Reflection in action – reflecting during the experience in a way that previous learning is used to improve practice at that moment in time.

Structured reflection

To be useful or action focused reflection has to be a structured process. There are a number of models available and most have a common structure (Figure 37.1) such as:
• Identifying and describing the experience/s.
• Examining the experience in depth, teasing out the key issues – what did I think at the time? how did I feel?

• Processing the issues – how do the issues relate to practice? what have I learnt?
• In the light of examining this experience, what actions do I need to take? how can I improve my practice?
     Learning to reflect in a structured way is important but it should not be used as a rigid formula; instead it should be used as a guide. It is also important to recognise that over time reflection on action if used properly as a lifelong learning tool will become more refined; it will also enable the nurse to reflect in action and also assist them towards being an expert practitioner.

Clinical supervision

Clinical supervision as a reflective practice can be delivered in different ways; these include:
• individual supervision;
• group supervision;
• peer group supervision.
Though it follows the tenets of structured reflection it can be grounded in a specific model, especially in the case of a mental health nurse who is also a therapist such as a cognitive behavioural therapist. Whatever model is used in clinical supervision, as a professional process it should:
• Support practice and enable the nurse to maintain and promote standards of care.
• Be a practice-focused professional relationship involving a practitioner reflecting on practice guided by a skilled supervisor.
• Be developed by practitioners and managers according to local circumstances; ground rules should be agreed so that practitioners and supervisors approach clinical supervision openly, confidently and are aware of what is involved.
• Ensure all practitioners should have access to clinical supervision and each supervisor should supervise a realistic number of practitioners.
• Confirm supervisors are adequately prepared, with the principles and relevance of clinical supervision being included in pre- and post-registration education programmes.
• Ensure that the practice of clinical supervision is evaluated locally with a focus on evaluating how it influences care, practice standards and the service.

Further reading

Jasper, M. & Rolfe, G. (2011) Critical reflection and the emergence of professional knowledge. In: Rolfe, G., Jasper, M. & Freshwater, D. (2011) *Critical Reflection in Practice: Generating Knowledge for Care*, 2nd edn. Basingstoke: Palgrave Macmillan, pp. 1–10.

Kedge, S. & Appleby, B. (2009) Promoting a culture of curiosity within nursing practice. *British Journal of Nursing* **18**(10): 635–7.

Schon, D. (1983) *The Reflective Practitioner: How Professionals Think in Action*. London: Temple Smith.

38 Lifelong learning

Figure 38.1 The practice tree: Lifelong learning

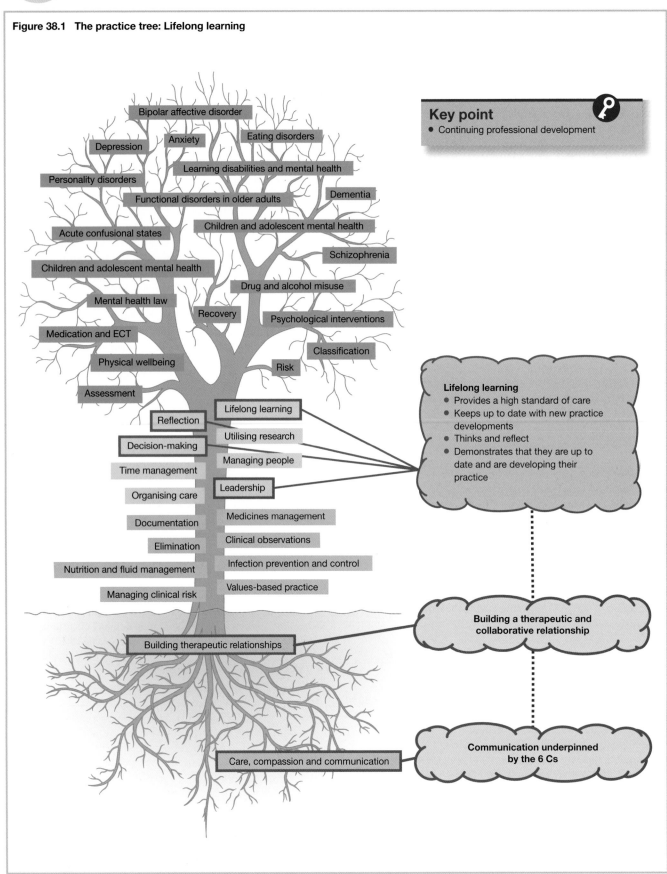

Introduction

Professionally mental health nurses should be committed lifelong learners who utilise the reflective process to explore, appreciate and develop their practice experiences. Continuing professional development is a key part of the nurse's lifelong learning journey, but lifelong learning is a wider concept that also takes into account personal learning, which or may not relate to a nurse's professional practice. Both these processes when actively underpinned by effective reflective practices will assist the nurse towards being an expert in their practice with the benefit of improving the care they deliver. It is important to recognise that as each nurse's experiences are unique then their lifelong learning journey will also be unique and dynamic. Being unique does not mean that formal education has no part to play in this journey; it just means that formal and informal learning should be utilised in ways that complement each other.

Competencies

Mental health nurses are required to:
- Through continuing professional development keep their knowledge and skills up to date by learning from experience, through supervision, feedback, reflection and evaluation.
- Demonstrate a commitment to their own and others' lifelong learning and professional development.
- Facilitate others, including nursing students, to develop their competence, using a range of professional and personal development skills.
- As team member and team leader, actively seek and learn from feedback to enhance care delivery.

The context

Lifelong learning is a commonly used term; it is broad in scope, referring to a process that takes place across an individual's lifespan and includes both formal and informal learning. In terms of mental health nursing the concept is used as an expectation that mental health nurses will keep their skills and knowledge up to date throughout their working lives. More formally and at a professional level, lifelong learning is entwined with the process of continuing professional development. On this basis the NMC has set a number of continuing professional development standards for post-registration education and practice (Prep) standards. These standards aim (see Figure 38.1) to assist the mental health nurse to:
- provide a high standard of care;
- keep up to date with new practice developments;
- think and reflect;
- demonstrate that they are up to date and are developing their practice.

Prep

The Prep standards are legal requirements set by the NMC that the nurse must adhere to in order to maintain and renew their registration. There are two standards articulated in the NMC's *The Prep Handbook* (2011) as follows:

- The practice standard requires the nurse to have practised in some capacity by virtue of their nursing qualification for a minimum of 450 hours during the three years prior to the renewal of their registration. If the nurse does not meet this requirement, they will need to undertake an approved return to practice course before they can renew their registration.
- The continuing professional development standard includes a commitment to undertake continuing professional development (CPD). The CPD standard requires the nurse to undertake at least 35 hours of learning activity relevant to their practice during the three years prior to renewal of registration; maintain a personal professional profile of their learning activity; and comply with any request from the NMC to audit how they have met these requirements.

Expert practice

By the mental health nurse engaging in maintaining and continually improving their practice they are engendering an opportunity to develop their expertise. The benefit of being an expert mental health nurse is that they are more effective than novice nurses when managing clinical situations that are ambiguous, complex and have no certain outcome. This does not mean that the novice nurse or newly qualified mental health nurse will not be able to cope with a range of situations it is just that at first they will not be as fluid in dealing with situations as the expert nurse. The knowledge and wide range of skills of the expert nurse are built through the nurse passing through a number of stages in their development; these stages (Figure 38.1) are described by the work of Benner (1982) and include:

1 Learning to be a registered nurse (novice).
2 Starting to use practical experiences to contextualise their knowledge.
3 Managing standard clinical situations but lacking speed and flexibility.
4 Recognising and understanding non-standard situations.
5 Not relying just on rules to manage situations but also using both scientific and naturalistic knowledge (expert).

Key to being an expert is the use of reflection. This process enables the nurse to develop their self-awareness to a level where they are able to clearly identify their strengths and also the areas that they need to develop further. It is important to recognise that knowledge accrued through the reflective process is useful knowledge especially as it is experience-based knowledge. Like scientific knowledge this form of knowledge should not be used in isolation; rather it should be used to complement scientific knowledge in a way that anchors both forms of knowledge to the nurse's ongoing practice experiences.

Further reading

Benner, P. (1982) From novice to expert. *The American Journal of Nursing* **82**(3): 402–7.

Person, H. (2009) Transition from nursing student to staff nurse: a personal reflection. *Paediatric Nursing* **21**(3): 30–2.

Smith, G. (2012) Conclusion: psychological interventions and the mental health nurse's future development. In: Smith, G. (ed.) *Psychological Interventions in Mental Health Nursing*. Maidenhead: Open University Press, pp. 155–64.

Appendix: Clinical procedures

Taking a pulse

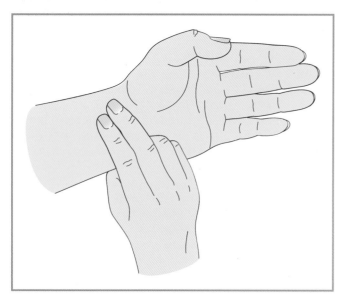

Appendix Figure 1   Taking a pulse.

Taking a blood pressure

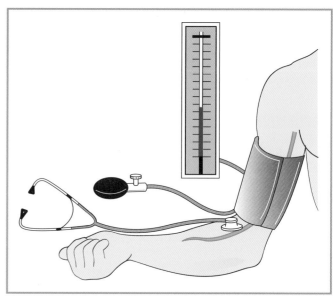

Appendix Figure 2   Checking blood pressure.

Context
See Chapter 8 – pulse section.

The nurse measures the pulse by "lightly compressing the artery against firm tissue and by counting the number of beats per minute" (Dougherty & Lister, 2011: p. 708). The pulse can also be measured electronically or by using a stethoscope to listen to the heart. Manually the pulse is usually measured at the radial site, located on the inside of the wrist near the side of the thumb, or at the carotid site, found on the neck between the wind pipe and neck muscle, just under the lower jaw bone.

Equipment
When measuring the pulse manually you will require:
- a watch with a second hand;
- alcohol hand rub.

Procedure
First of all you will need to explain the procedure to the service user and obtain their consent. Then you will need to:
- Wash your hands.
- Ensure the service user is comfortable and has refrained from physical activity for 20 minutes prior to their pulse being taken.
- Place the first and second finger along the artery and apply light pressure until the pulse is felt.
- Count the pulse (beats) for 60 seconds.
- Wash your hands.
- Document the results and report any unexpected readings.

Context
See Chapter 8 – blood pressure section.

In terms of methods of measuring blood pressure this can be done manually or through the use of an automated machine. Blood pressure can also be measured continuously such as where a service user is critically ill, or it can be measured intermittently. Usually blood pressure is measured at the brachial artery but in some cases alternative sites can be used.

Equipment
When measuring blood pressure manually and at the brachial site you will require:
- an appropriately sized cuff;
- a calibrated sphygmomanometer;
- stethoscope;
- chair with an arm rest or equivalent;
- detergent hand wipes.

Procedure
Firstly you will need to explain the procedure to the service user and obtain their consent. Then you will need to:
- Wash your hands.
- Check that there are no problems with using a particular arm.
- Ensure the service user is seated and rests for three to five minutes before taking their blood pressure. They should not be eating, drinking or talking when their blood pressure measurement is taken.
- Ensure that the upper arm is supported and positioned at heart level, and is free from clothing. The manometer should be no more than a metre away and it should be at eye level.

Mental Health Nursing at a Glance, First Edition. Grahame Smith. © 2015 John Wiley & Sons, Ltd. Published 2015 by John Wiley & Sons, Ltd.
Companion website: www.ataglanceseries.com/nursing/mentalhealth

- Wrap the cuff around the arm ensuring that the centre of the bladder covers the brachial artery.
- Inflate the cuff while palpating the brachial artery. When the pulse can no longer be felt rapidly inflate the cuff for a further 20–30 mmHg.
- Deflate the cuff until the pulse reappears; note the reading and then deflate the cuff.
- After 15–20 seconds place the diaphragm of the stethoscope over the brachial artery; do not tuck the diaphragm under the edge of the cuff.
- Inflate the cuff again to 20– 30 mmHg of the first reading.
- Deflate the cuff at 2–3 mmHg per second or per heartbeat until the first tapping sounds (first of the Korotkoff sounds) are heard; note the reading – systolic blood pressure.
- Continue to deflate the cuff slowly until the Korotkoff sounds disappear (usually the fifth Korotkoff sound); note this reading – the best representation of diastolic blood pressure.
- Once no further sounds can be heard rapidly deflate the cuff.
- Wash your hands and clean the bell of the stethoscope and cuff with the hand wipes.
- Document the results and report any unexpected readings.

Measuring respiration

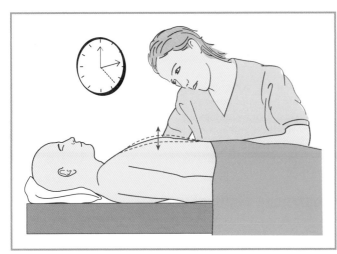

Appendix Figure 3   Measuring respiration.

Context
See Chapter 8 – respiratory rate section.

Equipment
When measuring respiration rate you will require:
- a watch with a second hand.

Procedure
Firstly you will need to explain the procedure to the service user and obtain their consent. Then you will need to:
- Ensure the patient is comfortable.
- To avoid the service user altering their breathing monitor and record their respirations immediately after taking the pulse.
- Observe the rise (inspiration) and fall of the chest (expiration) – one breath.
- Count the service user's respirations for 60 seconds.
- Also note the pattern of breathing and the depth of the service user's breath.
- Document the results and report any unexpected readings.

Measuring peak flow

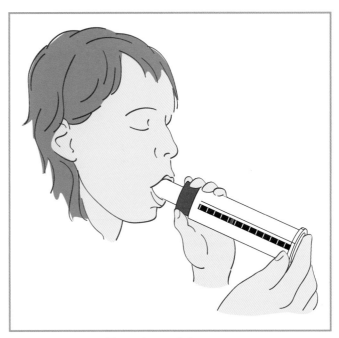

Appendix Figure 4   Measuring peak flow.

Context
This is measuring the "maximum flow of air which can be achieved when air is expired with maximum force following maximum inspiration" (Dougherty & Lister, 2011: p. 745).

Equipment
When measuring peak flow you will require:
- a calibrated peak flow meter;
- disposable mouthpiece.

Procedure
Firstly you will need to explain the procedure to the service user and obtain their consent. Then you will need to:
- Wash your hands.
- Assemble the peak flow meter using a clean mouthpiece.
- Ask the service user to adopt a comfortable position, which can be either sitting or standing. The same position should be used for future readings.
- Set the pointer on the scale to zero.
- Ask the service user to hold the peak flow meter horizontally.
- Ask the service user to take a deep breath (full inspiration) through their mouth.
- Ask the service user to place their lips tightly around the mouthpiece, ensuring a good seal; the inspiration should not be held longer than 2 seconds.
- Ask the service user to breathe out as hard and as fast as possible.
- Note the reading, and then ask the service user to repeat the procedure twice.
- Document the results and report any unexpected or abnormal readings.
- Dispose of the mouthpiece and clean the meter.
- Wash your hands.

Measuring temperature

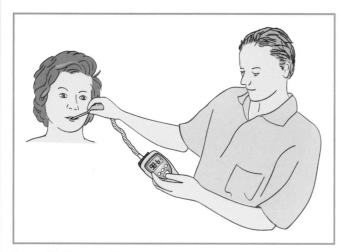

Appendix Figure 5   Measuring temperature.

Context

See Chapter 8 – temperature section.

Temperature can be measured at a number of sites; historically the mouth, axilla and rectum have been the preferred sites. With the development of new technology it is now more common to measure temperature via the tympanic membrane or ear canal (Dougherty & Lister, 2011).

Equipment

When measuring the temperature (tympanic membrane) you will require:

- tympanic membrane thermometer;
- disposable probe covers;
- alcohol hand rub.

Procedure

Firstly you will need to explain the procedure to the service user and obtain their consent. Then you will need to:

- Wash your hands.
- Ensure you have good access to the service user's ear and document which ear is being used – consistency of results.
- Apply the disposable cover.
- Place the probe gently into the ear.
- Measure the temperature and record the reading.
- Dispose of the probe cover.
- Wash your hands.
- Document the results and report any unexpected readings.

Undertaking a urinalysis (dipstick testing)

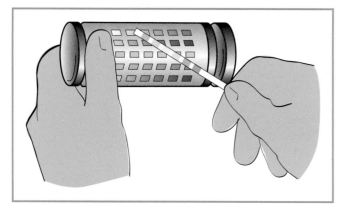

Appendix Figure 6   Dipstick testing.

Context

Urinalysis is where the physical, chemical and microscopic properties of urine are analysed (Dougherty & Lister, 2011). Nurses would commonly analyse urine through the use of "dipstick" tests. This is where a strip coated with chemicals is dipped into urine and the results are compared with the manufacturer's guidelines, which are usually on the bottle or container (Dougherty & Lister, 2011).

Equipment

When undertaking a "dipstick" test you will require:

- gloves;
- apron;
- urine dipsticks that are in date and have not been contaminated;
- urine specimen bottle.

Procedure

Firstly you will need to explain the procedure to the service user and obtain their consent. Then you will need to:

- Wash your hands and put on your gloves and apron.
- Collect a clean and fresh specimen of urine.
- Remove the dipstick and immediately replace the cap on the container.
- Immerse the dipstick into urine and wait for the appropriate length of time.
- Run the edge of the strip against the rim of the specimen bottle to remove any excess urine.
- Hold dipstick at a slight angle, preventing pad-to-pad contamination.
- After waiting the required length of time compare the strip against the reference guide on the dipstick container.
- Dispose of urine and dipstick.
- Remove gloves and apron.
- Wash your hands.
- Document the results and report any abnormal readings.

Measuring blood glucose

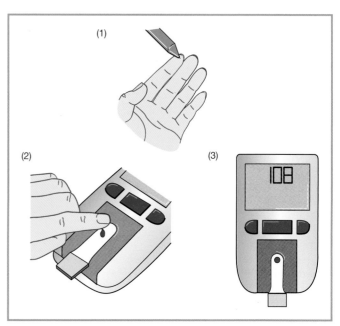

Appendix Figure 7   Measuring blood glucose.

Context

This is measuring the amount of glucose in the blood, which is expressed as millimoles per litre (mmol/L); the normal range is 4–8 mmol/L (Dougherty & Lister, 2011).

Equipment

You will require:

- a calibrated blood glucose meter/monitor;
- test strips that are in date and have not been contaminated;
- single-use lancets and lancet device;
- gloves;
- cotton wool or similar;
- sharps box.

Procedure

Firstly you will need to explain the procedure to the service user and obtain their consent. Then you will need to:

- Ask the service-user to either sit or lie down.
- Wash your hands and then put on your gloves.
- Insert a clean lancet into the lancet device.
- Using an appropriate lancet depth and remembering to rotate the piercing site take a blood sample from the side of the finger.
- Apply a drop of blood to the correct part of the testing strip.
- Place the strip in the meter; some meters may require that you place the strip in the meter before taking a sample of blood.
- Dispose of the lancet in the sharps box.
- Place the cotton wool or gauze over the puncture site and apply gentle pressure if required; monitor for excessive bleeding.
- Follow the monitor directions to obtain a reading.
- Wash your hands.
- Document the results and report any unexpected readings, errors or excessive bleeding.

References and bibliography

Bach, S. & Ellis, P. (2011) *Leadership, Management and Team Working in Nursing*. Exeter: Learning Matters.

Baker, P. (ed.) (2009) *Psychiatric and Mental Health Nursing: The Craft of Caring,* 2nd edn. London: Hodder Arnold.

Callaghan, P., Playle, J. & Cooper, L. (eds) (2009) *Mental Health Nursing Skills*. Oxford: Oxford University Press.

Commissioning Board Chief Nursing Officer and DH Chief Nursing Adviser (2012) *Compassion in Practice*. London: DH and the NHS Commissioning Board.

Davey, G. (2008) *Psychopathology: Research, Assessment and Treatment in Clinical Psychology*. Oxford: Wiley-Blackwell.

Dougherty, L. & Lister, S. (eds) (2011) *The Royal Marsden Hospital Manual of Clinical Nursing Procedures: Student Edition*, 8th edn. Chichester: Wiley-Blackwell.

Harris, N., Baker, J. & Gray, R. (eds) (2009) *Medicines Management in Mental Health Care*. Chichester: Wiley-Blackwell.

Katona, C., Cooper, C. & Robertson, M. (2012) *Psychiatry at a Glance*, 5th edn. Oxford: Wiley-Blackwell.

Nash, M. (2010) *Physical Health and Well-Being in Mental Health Nursing: Clinical Skills for Practice*. Maidenhead: Open University Press.

Norman, I. & Ryrie, I. (eds) (2013) *The Art and Science of Mental Health Nursing: Principles and Practice*, 3rd edn. Maidenhead: Open University Press.

Northern Ireland Practice and Education Council (2010) *Evidencing Care: Improving Record Keeping Practice a Guide on Care Planning*. Belfast: NIPEC.

Nursing and Midwifery Council (2008) Advice Sheet: Clinical Supervision. London: NMC.

Nursing and Midwifery Council (2008) *Standards for Medicines Management*. London: NMC.

Nursing and Midwifery Council (2009) *Record Keeping: Guidance for Nurses and Midwives*. London: NMC.

Nursing and Midwifery Council (2010) *Standards for Pre-registration Nursing Education*. London: NMC.

Nursing and Midwifery Council (2011) *The Prep handbook*. London: NMC.

O'Carroll, M. & Park, A. (2007) *Essential Mental Health Nursing Skills*. London, Mosby.

Rolfe, G., Jasper, M. & Freshwater, D. (2011) *Critical Reflection in Practice: Generating Knowledge for Care*, 2nd edn. Basingstoke: Palgrave Macmillan.

Smith, G. (ed.) (2012) *Psychological Interventions in Mental Health Nursing*. Maidenhead: Open University Press.

Standing Nursing and Midwifery Advisory Committee (1999) Practice guidance: Safe and supportive observation of patients at risk mental health nursing – Addressing acute concerns. London: DH.

Thompson, N. (2009) *People Skills*, 3rd edn. Basingstoke: Palgrave Macmillan.

Wright, P. (2006) *Core Psychopharmacology*. London: Saunders Elsevier.

Glossary

abstinence: Supporting an individual to refrain from using a drug and/or alcohol.

acute detoxification: Supporting an individual to rapidly withdraw from an addictive substance.

adjustment disorders: Where an individual finds it difficult to adjust or cope with an identifiable life event.

administering medication: One can administer non-prescribed medication and/or illicit medication.

amenorrhoea: The absence of menstrual periods.

apathy: Lack of interest, emotion, or concern.

art therapy: Using art as a therapy to deal with difficult emotions in a healthy way.

assessment: Establishing an understanding of a service user's situation through a process of asking questions.

assessment methods: Using checklists, questionnaires, rating scales, tools, structured interviews, day-to-day observations and interactions.

authoritarian team leader: One who adopts predominantly an autocratic style of leadership.

autonomy: The ability and freedom to self-govern.

balanced diet: Eating the right amounts of certain food groups.

behavioural activation: Utilising reinforcement to influence the development of desired behaviours.

behavioural therapy: A range of behavioural techniques that focus on reinforcing desired behaviours.

blood pressure: The force of blood or pressure against the vessel walls.

Body Mass Index (BMI): Indicator of bodyweight, calculated as body mass (kg) divided by the square of the individual's height (m).

bradycardia: Slow heart rate.

cannabis: A drug that that can have a "relaxing" effect but individuals can also experience confusion, hallucinations, anxiety and paranoia.

Care Programme Approach (CPA): A risk management process within the field of mental health.

case studies: A descriptive exploration of an individual or an individual's circumstances.

catatonic: A disorder of motor function where an individual may remain still for long periods of time.

classification: Identifying, grouping and ordering mental disorders.

clinical governance: A process whereby healthcare organisations improve the quality of the services they provide.

clinical observations (vital signs): Temperature, pulse, respiratory rate and blood pressure.

cognitive restructuring: Identifying and changing irrational thoughts.

cognitive stimulation: A brief psychological treatment for individuals diagnosed with mild to moderate dementia that focuses on providing structured activities that are cognitively stimulating.

collaboration: Working together within the therapeutic relationship.

communication: A two-way process that requires the effective use of verbal and non-verbal communication skills.

coping strategy work: An individual is supported to develop healthy coping strategies.

Creutzfeldt–Jakob disease: A degenerative and fatal disorder of the brain that is progressive and quickly leads to dementia.

delusion: A fixed, false belief.

desensitisation: A process of reducing sensitivity by repeated and supported exposure to a difficult situation or stimulus.

diagnosis: An assessment process that focuses on collecting information and formulating a treatment plan.

dialectic behaviour therapy: Supporting individuals diagnosed with a borderline personality disorder to cope with emotional difficulties in a healthy way.

documentation: Record keeping.

domains: The required knowledge, skills and attitudes a student nurse needs to attain to qualify; these include professional values, communication and interpersonal skills, nursing practice and decision-making, and leadership, management and team working.

DSM: *Diagnostic and Statistical Manual of Mental Disorders.*

electroencephalography (EEG): Measuring the electrical activity of the brain.

elimination: Bowel and bladder habits.

empathetic: Being an active listener, genuinely interested, accepting the person and being caring and compassionate.

empathy: Being able to identify with the service user's experiences.

encopresis: Voluntary or involuntary soiling.

enuresis: Inability to control urination usually at night time.

ethical practice: Utilising the relevant ethical theories, understanding the relevant professional rules, and also having the skills to ethically reason.

ethical reasoning: A systematic process underpinned by an ethical framework.

Ethical theories: Theories that focus on what actions are right, what ought to be done, what motives are good, and what characteristics are virtuous.

ethnography: A research method that focuses on studying and exploring cultural living.

family therapy: A therapy that focuses on working with families and couples.

field skills: The knowledge, skills and attitudes that nurses must acquire in order to practise in a specific field of nursing.

fields of nursing: Formerly known as branches of nursing, includes four fields: mental health, adult, child and learning disabilities.

focus group: A research method that explores the opinions, beliefs and attitudes of a group of individuals.

generic skills: The knowledge, skills and attitudes required of all nurses by the end of a pre-registration nursing programme.

Grade Exposure and Response Prevention: Supporting an individual to confront their obsessions in a structured way.

grounded theory: Discovering theory through the research process.

group therapy: Psychological therapies within a group setting.

guided self-help: A problem-focused approach that assists individuals to change the way they think, feel and behave.

hallucination: A perception of the outside world that is perceived as being true even though there is no external stimulus; for example, hearing a voice when no one is there.

hallucinogens: A group of drugs that disrupt an individual's sense of reality.

harm reduction strategies: Supporting an individual to learn practical strategies that reduce the harms associated with drug use.

health promotion: At an individual level focuses on enabling individuals to control and improve their health and wellbeing.

Huntington's disease: A degenerative and genetic disorder of the brain that is characterised by muscle incoordination and cognitive and mental health difficulties.

hyperkinetic disorders: A behavioural syndrome usually seen in children where the individual is hyperactive, impulsive and finds it difficult to concentrate.

hypoglycaemia: Low blood sugar.

hypothermia: A body temperature reading below 35.0 °C.

ICD: International Classification of Diseases.

incontinence: An inability to control the function of the bladder or bowel.

infection control and prevention: A zero tolerance of infection.

Mental Health Nursing at a Glance, First Edition. Grahame Smith. © 2015 John Wiley & Sons, Ltd. Published 2015 by John Wiley & Sons, Ltd.
Companion website: www.ataglanceseries.com/nursing/mentalhealth

infection control skills: Effective infection prevention and control practices and techniques.

interpersonal therapy: A time-limited psychological therapy that supports an individual to healthily control their mood and emotions within the context of their everyday relationships.

medication adherence: Taking medication as prescribed.

mental distress: Metal health problems that cannot be fully captured by using the term mental illness.

mental health nursing practice tree: An illustrative guide to the mental health nurse making reasoned decisions.

mentalisation-based approaches: Supporting individuals diagnosed with a borderline personality disorder to recognise and understand the relationship between their actions and their mental states.

mindfulness approaches: Supporting the individual to focus their attention and awareness.

Motivational Enhancement Therapy: Support for individuals to engage in treatment for their drug and/or alcohol use.

Motivational Interviewing: A psychological approach that focuses on supporting the individual to change specific behaviours.

narrative studies: Systematically studying the effective elements of individuals' stories.

NMC: Nursing and Midwifery Council.

NMC's Code of Conduct: A professional code that nurses are required to adhere to.

normal temperature: A body temperature reading between 36.0 and 37.2 °C.

nutritional support: Assisting the service user to meet their nutritional needs.

opiates: A class of drugs that depress the central nervous system.

Parkinson's disease: A degenerative disorder of the nervous system characterised by movement problems.

personality: An individual's thinking, feeling and behaving patterns, which are either viewed as unique to the individual or seen as being measurable through identifying personality traits.

pharmacological: Describing the actions, uses and effects of drug treatments.

phenomenology: Focuses on studying an individual's conscious understanding of a given experience.

Pick's disease: A degenerative disorder of the brain that is characterised by speech, cognitive and behavioural difficulties.

positive risk management: A risk management approach that is collaborative and recovery focused.

pre-therapy work: Helping prepare individuals to engage with psychological therapies.

professional boundaries: Adhering within the NMC's professional code of conduct.

professional competencies: Competencies that mental health nursing students are professionally required to attain before they qualify.

psychoeducation: Education about an individual's condition and how to manage their symptoms.

psychological interventions: Mental health nursing interventions underpinned by psychological methods and theory with the intention of improving biopsychosocial functioning

psychosocial interventions: Types of psychological interventions.

pulse: The measurement of an individual's heart rate.

pyrexia: A body temperature reading above 37.5 °C.

Reality Orientation Therapy: A therapy that focuses on reducing confusion, disorientation and memory loss through orienting the individual to the present time, place and person.

resilience: An individual's ability to cope with psychosocial adversity.

respiratory rate: The rate, rhythm and depth of breathing.

risk: Adverse incidents that are waiting to happen.

risk management: A systematic process that focuses on managing identified risk.

risk management – mental health care: Managing the likelihood that harm to self and/or others will occur.

social learning strategies: Supporting an individual to learn from others' (society) healthy coping strategies that can be used within a social context.

solution-focused Therapy: A brief psychological therapy that is goal-oriented and focuses on present and future solutions rather than looking at past problems.

stimulants: A class of drugs that stimulate the central nervous system.

strengths model: Focusing on the strengths of the individual and their circumstances as a way to aid recovery.

stroke: Also known as a cerebrovascular accident, is where brain function is adversely affected due to the blood supply being cut off to a part or parts of the brain.

structured physical activity: Promoting physical activity in a planned way for older adults.

suicide: Intentional self-inflicted death.

supportive observations: Levels of observation that are utilised as risk management interventions in the field of mental health nursing.

Systemic Therapy: A therapy that is concerned with individuals and their relationships and interactions within a group context.

tachycardia: An abnormally fast "resting" heart rate.

Therapeutic Community Treatments: Using a residential group-based approach to treat individuals diagnosed with personality disorders or drug and alcohol problems.

therapeutic relationship: A professional relationship between the mental health nurse and the service that is partnership focused, person centred and non-discriminatory.

therapeutic self: The nurse being self-aware and using this knowledge in a positive way when working with service users.

The 6 Cs: Six core communication skills within a nursing context Care, Compassion, Competence, Communication, Courage and Commitment.

Validation Therapy: A psychological approach that focuses on respecting the person through the use of structured communication.

values-based practice: A process focusing on managing ethical conflict within the mental health practice field.

vascular dementia: Dementia caused by vascular problems, which can result in the individual having a series of mini-strokes that adversely affect brain function.

volition: Desire or will.

Index

'6 Cs' 3

acute confusional states 52–3
adolescents 56–7
Adults with Incapacity Act 2000 63
ageing process 49
alcohol misuse 54–5
alcohol use 55
Alzheimer's disease 51
anorexia nervosa 43
antidementia drugs 69
antidepressants 67
antipsychotics 67
anxiety 40–1, 67
  in older adults 49
anxiolytics 67
assessment 24–5
  see also physical health assessment;
    risk assessment
assessment skills 25
assessment tools 25

benzodiazepines 67
best practice 73
binge drinking 55
binge eating disorder 43
bipolar affective disorder 38–9, 67
bladder care 15
Bleuler, Paul Eugen 35
blood glucose 90–1
blood pressure 17, 88–9
body language 3
bowel care 15
bulimia nervosa 43
buspirone 67

carbamazepine 69
care 2–3
  delivery 25, 73
  organising 72–3
  person-centred 73
Care Programme Approach (CPA) 27
case management approach 73
change 77
children 56–7, 69
classification 28–30
clinical governance 9
clinical leadership 75
clinical observations 16–17
clinical supervision 85
closed questions 25
coaching 77
code of conduct 5, 7
collaboration 33
communication 2–3
Community Treatment Order (CTO) 65
compassion 2–3
consequentialism 7
constipation 15
continuing professional
  development (CPD) 87
critical reflection 5, 33, 84–5, 87

decision-making 80–1
delegation 79
delirium 53
dementia 50–1, 69
dementia praecox 35

deontology 7
depression 36–7, 53, 67
  and physical health problems 61
  in older adults 49
diagnosis 30
Diagnostic and Statistical Manual
  of Mental Disorders (DSM) 30
diet 13
dipstick testing see urinalysis
documentation 18–19
donepezil 69
drug misuse 54–5

eating disorders 42–3
ECT see electroconvulsive therapy
electroconvulsive therapy (ECT) 66–9
elimination 14–15
empathy 5
Enduring Powers of Attorney
  Order 1987 63
essential skills 1–21
ethical conflict 7
ethical reasoning 7
ethical theory 7
evidence 83
evidence-based interventions 5, 33
evidence-based knowledge 81
evidence-based practice (EBP) 83
experience-based knowledge 87
expert practice 87

fluid management 12–13
functional disorders 48–9

generalised anxiety disorder (GAD) 41

harmful drinking 55
hazardous drinking 55
hazards 9
holistic assessments 25
holistic care 32, 62, 67, 73
holistic competencies xiii
Human Rights Act 1998 63
hypertension 17
hypnotics 67
hypotension 17
hypothermia 17

incontinence 15
infections
  prevention and control 10–11
  spreading of 11
International Classification
  of Diseases (ICD) 30

Jaspers, Karl 29

Kantianism 7
knowledge
  evidence-based 81
  experience-based 87
  types of 83
Kraepelin, Emil 29, 35

leadership 74–5
  models of 75
leadership skills 71–87
learning disabilities 46–7
lifelong learning 86–7

listening 3
lithium 67, 69

management 75
mania 53
manic depression see bipolar
  affective disorder
medication
  and ECT 66–9
  management 20–1
memantine 69
Mental Act Commission 65
Mental Capacity Act 2005
  (England and Wales) 63–4
mental distress 29
Mental Health Act (MHA) 1983
  (England and Wales) 63–5
Mental Health (Care and Treatment)
  (Scotland) Act 2003 64–5
Mental Health Commission 65
mental health law 62–5
Mental Health (Northern Ireland)
  Order 1986 65
mental retardation see learning
  disabilities
Mental Welfare Commission 65
mentoring 77
meta-communication 3
mood stabilisers 67–9

naturalistic evidence 83
neurocognitive disorders (NCD) 51
non-verbal communication 3
Nursing and Midwifery Council
  (NMC) 7, 19, 21, 87
nutrition 12–13

obsessive compulsive disorder
  (OCD) 41
older adults 48–9
  and delirium 53
'open dialogue' approach 33
open questions 3, 25
organizational culture 9

panic disorder 41
paralanguage 3
patient specific direction (PSD) 21
people management 76–7
personality disorders 44–5
person-centred care 73
person-centred philosophy 5
phobia 41
physical health 61
physical health assessment 61
physical health interventions 11
physical wellbeing 60–1
post-registration education and practice
  (Prep) 87
post-traumatic stress disorder
  (PTSD) 41
practice evidence 83
practice tree xiii–xv
Prep see post-registration education
  and practice
primary nursing approach 73
principlism 7
probing questions 3, 25

professional boundaries 5
psychological interventions 31–3
  anxiety 41
  bipolar affective disorder 39
  children and adolescents 57
  delirium 53
  dementia 51
  depression 37
  drug and alcohol misuse 55
  eating disorders 43
  in older adults 49
  learning disabilities 47
  personality disorders 45
  schizophrenia 35
psychological therapies 32 see also
  psychological interventions
psychosis 67
psychotic disorders 35
pulse 17, 88
pyrexia 17

real-time decisions 81
record keeping 19
recovery 58–9
recovery-based approach 59
recovery process 59
reflection see critical reflection
research, utilising 82–3
respiratory rate 17, 89
responding 3
risk 5, 9, 26–7
  and organizational culture 9
  dynamic 27
  static 27
risk assessment 27
risk management 8–9, 27
rivastigmine 69

schizophrenia 34–5, 53
scientific evidence 83
self-disclosure 5
self-harm 57
service-user allocation approach 73
sodium valproate 69
stress 79
substance misuse 55
supportive observations 27

task approach 73
team nursing approach 73
temperature 17, 90
therapeutic relationships 4–5
therapeutic self 5
tidal model 59
time management 78–9

urinalysis 90
utilitarianism 7

values-based practice 6–7
verbal communication 3
virtue ethics 7
vocals 3

weight gain 13

zolpidem 67
zopiclone 67

Mental Health Nursing at a Glance, First Edition. Grahame Smith. © 2015 John Wiley & Sons, Ltd. Published 2015 by John Wiley & Sons, Ltd.
Companion website: www.ataglanceseries.com/nursing/mentalhealth